we can all eat that!

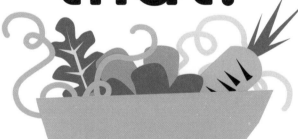

Dedication

This book is dedicated to paediatric allergist Dr Velencia Soutter MBBS FRACP (Paed). If it wasn't for her there wouldn't be a book. Sadly Velencia died in late 2019 and she is sorely missed by family, friends and her patients, to whom she gave so much.

A percentage of the profits go to the Velencia Soutter Memorial Fund at the Royal Prince Alfred Hospital in Sydney, for further research on, and treatment of, children's food allergies and intolerances.

Pam is also grateful for the advice of dietitian Dr Anne Swain, from the Royal Prince Alfred Hospital's Allergy Unit, who gave her advice and support on the completion of this book after Velencia's passing.

we can all eat that!

Raise healthy, adventurous eaters and help prevent food allergies

Pam Brook

with chefs Sarah Swan and Sam Gowing

Hardie Grant

BOOKS

contents

part one

Introducing food and food allergens to your baby

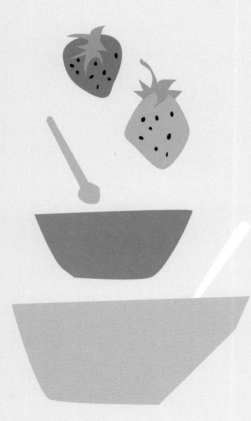

part two

The recipes

part three

Understanding food allergies and related conditions

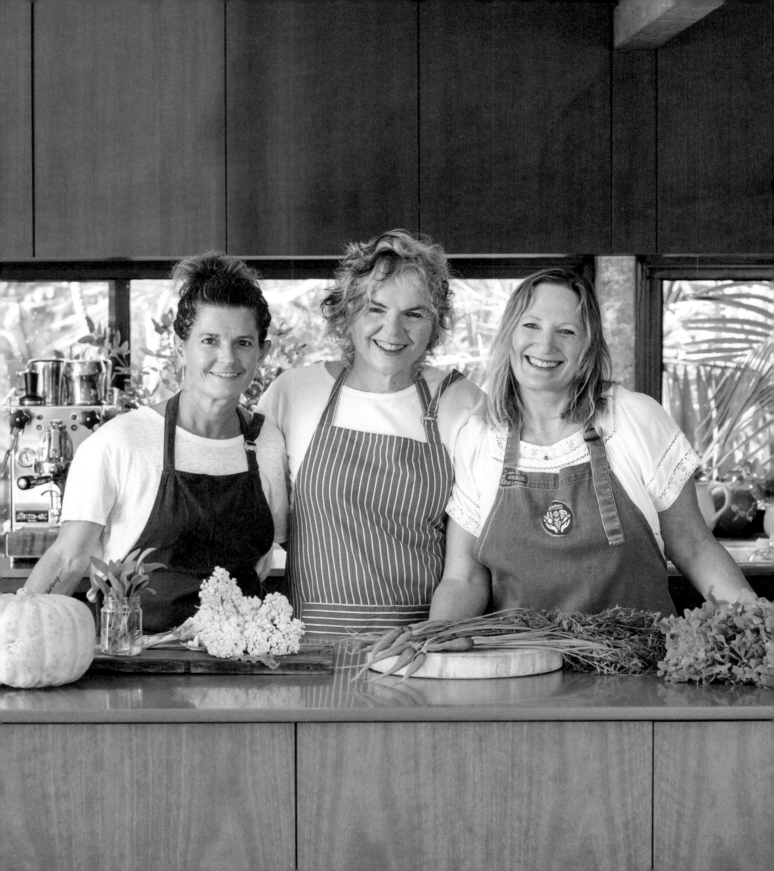

About the authors

Pam Brook

Born in Melbourne, Pam has a Bachelor of Dental Science from Melbourne University and a Master of Business Administration from Southern Cross University. Pam is co-founder of Brookfarm, a family food business based in Byron Bay, which she established with her husband, Martin Brook, on their macadamia farm in 1999. All their recipes began in Pam's kitchen, and Pam still creates all the new products today. She believes it's not enough for food to be healthy - it has to taste delicious, especially if you want your kids to eat it. She is passionate about nutritional balance, regenerative farming and 'real food made right'. She loves sharing and creating meals with family and friends.

Our chefs

SARAH SWAN One of Australia's great cooks and with more than 25 years' experience, Sarah's background stretches from The Bayswater Brasserie, Bathers' Pavilion and Rockpool in Sydney, to 100 Mile Table in Byron Bay. In 2019 Sarah turned her hand to retail and now owns and runs Bay Grocer in the heart of Byron. 100 Mile Table continues to thrive through its catering arm, as well as the food project at Stone & Wood Brewery. Sarah is passionate about provenance, and through her recipes she brings out the flavours of real ingredients. The art in her cooking is using simplicity to create fabulous, healthy, delicious food. Her uncompromising attention to detail and her understanding of produce and its origins is exceptional.

SAM GOWING Before nutrition became trendy, before kale became the superfood superstar, and before the green juice Instagram selfie was ever a thing, there was Sam Gowing, spreading the word on healthy cuisine and all that it encompasses. Sam is a chef's hat-winning restaurateur, who traded in her fast-paced city career to follow her passion for health and wellbeing. She retrained as a clinical nutritionist and more recently completed a master's degree with Le Cordon Bleu. Combining these skills with her celebrated cooking talents, Sam has established herself as one of Australia's leading nutritional chefs, kick-starting the 'food as medicine' movement, which is now a widely embraced philosophy around the world.

Why this book?

Today many families live in fear of food. Making decisions about what to feed your family can be challenging when you are inundated daily by the media and online, with often conflicting advice.

There is genuine concern around food allergies, which are on the rise. Although food allergies affect only a small percentage of children - about 4-8 per cent under the age of 5 - the concern for families today is that the number of children developing food allergies, especially peanut and tree-nut allergies, is continuing to rise significantly. It's not just the children of people who have allergies who are developing them, it's also children with no allergic history in their family.

The fear and frustration that families with food allergies live with every day requires constant vigilance, which can take its toll both physically and emotionally.

But is there a way to prevent food allergies?

Allergy experts from around the world now advise that early introduction of the common food allergens to children between the ages of 6 and 12 months may greatly reduce the risk of them developing an allergy to those foods.

By sharing the advice of allergy experts, this book hopes to help families be better informed about the common food allergens, their introduction to your child's diet from the very beginning, and when to seek expert advice and the appropriate precautions to take.

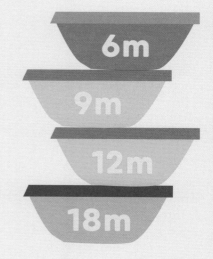

Early introduction of the common food allergens to children between the ages of 6 and 12 months may greatly reduce the risk of them developing an allergy to those foods

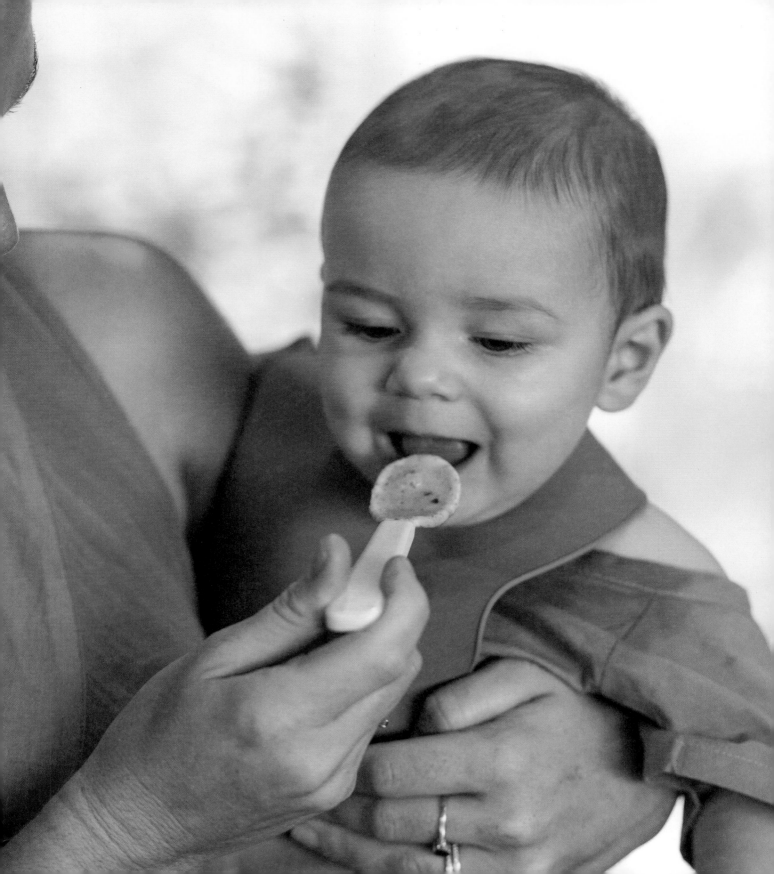

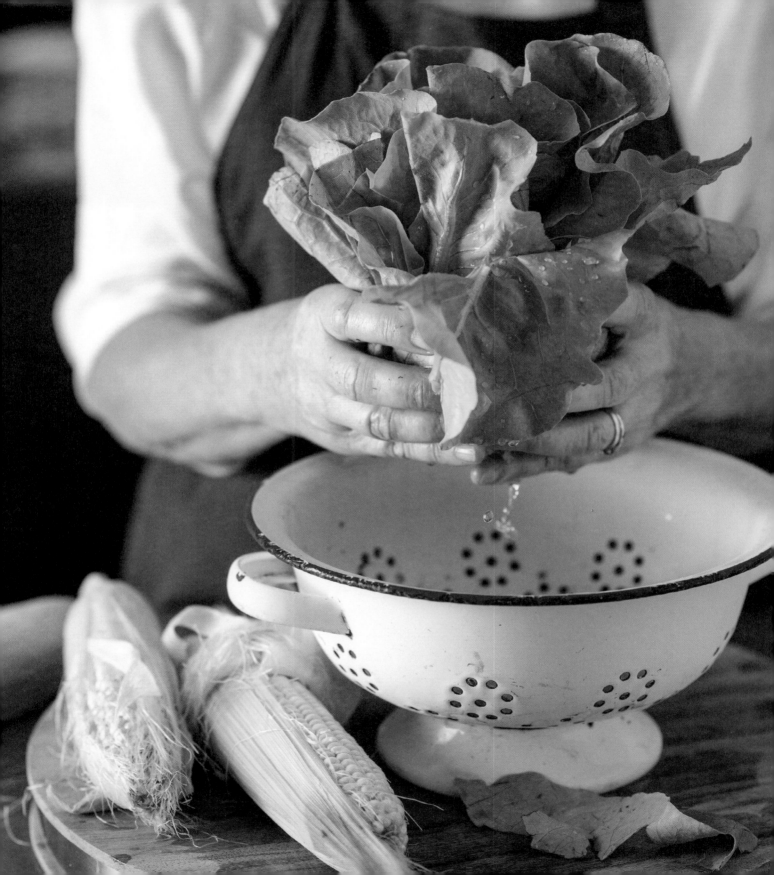

A nutrition journey

I grew up in Melbourne in the 1950s. My family rarely ate takeaway or processed foods, and we sat around the table for meals. It was an era when food allergies were hardly ever talked about or experienced. My mum was a great home cook - nothing flash, but she always used fresh ingredients. She made a mean apple pie with unpeeled apples. My dad lived fitness and good nutrition all his life, still climbing mountains and skiing in his 80s. Food was always at the centre of our family gatherings and celebrations. I was raised to love sharing home-cooked meals, and I've always enjoyed cooking, even when the results were less than spectacular. Now I'm the mother of two beautiful sons, Will and Eddie, who were also brought up with a love of real food cooked right.

My nutrition journey was different. I spent 25 years of my life as a dentist (and a working mum), treating children and families of all ages. In my dentist world, sugar intake was the biggest health problem I saw, and I thought I knew quite a bit about nutrition. Then a career switch to the food industry changed everything. I began to learn the stories behind where our food comes from. Our everyday food choices make a difference both to us and to the environment.

In 1999 my husband, Martin, and I became macadamia nut farmers with a passion to share the story of healthy, real food grown on regenerative farms. We wanted to introduce macadamia nuts to everyday foods, made the way I cook food - free from additives and preservatives and tasting delicious. Nut allergies weren't high on my radar at the time, but I was soon to learn about them.

REAL FOOD COOKED RIGHT

In this book we talk a lot about real food cooked right. This means cooking with fresh, unprocessed (preferably in-season) ingredients grown by farmers who care for their soils and the environment, and who grow pesticide-free and organic produce with better nutritional value. You'll find excellent fruit, vegetables and meats at farmers' markets and retailers who actually know their farmers. Real food could even come from your own garden and be as simple as fresh herbs grown in pots in your kitchen. It also means minimally processed foods crafted with care, such as soft and hard cheeses made using traditional methods, stocks and broths made without additives and preservatives, and delicious fermented foods such as yoghurt and sourdough bread. Food that is cooked right is delicious, nourishing and home-cooked using the very best produce you can afford.

The idea for this book was sparked when I met paediatric allergist Dr Velencia Soutter in April 2018. I had contacted Velencia to learn more about introducing the common food allergens in children's first foods, for a baby cereal I was developing. Velencia and I found we had so much in common - we discovered we shared a love of real food cooked at home and a passion for regenerative farming and rainforest restoration on our farms.

The world of a paediatric allergist was so foreign to me, and for the first time I better understood the fear that families with food allergies live with every day. Velencia inspired me to write this book, to take a serious look at the issues surrounding food allergies an d to encourage families to embrace home cooking and adventurous, healthy eating.

Most of all I wanted to make it easy for the whole family to eat the same meal, with just a few variations for babies or toddlers, rather than having to cook something different for everyone.

Food marketing is often more about what's left out, because 'free from' is perceived as safer. However, the result can be a lack of flavour and nutrients for your baby. Babies are not being introduced to the common allergens such as peanuts, tree nuts, eggs, dairy, wheat, sesame, soy and seafood due to fear of allergic reactions. However, allergy experts now advise that early introduction of the common allergy-causing foods to children between the ages of 6 and 12 months may greatly reduce the risk of them developing an allergy to those foods.

Whatever age we are - baby, toddler, teenager, or young or older adult - we all need to eat a healthy, balanced diet and look after our physical and mental wellbeing and fitness, whether we are allergy-free or managing allergies or other illnesses. It's time to get back to delicious home cooking. More than ever we need real food cooked right.

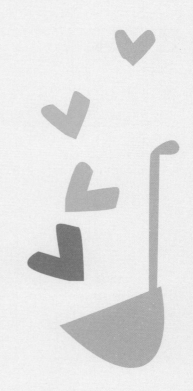

I wanted to make it easy for the whole family to eat the same meal, with just a few variations for babies or toddlers

How to use this book

This book is designed to help demystify children's first foods, give you insights into food allergies, and inspire you to create delicious home-cooked meals for the whole family.

Part One keeps it simple. Learn when your baby is ready for solids, how to introduce baby's first food and make easy, quick, healthy and delicious first meals at home. We introduce the common food allergens and the latest advice on their introduction.

Part Two is a recipe book unlike any other. It's a simple guide to preparing food for your baby and your family that provides variety and nutrition, and incorporates many of the common food allergens. We give you alternatives and flexibility, and show clearly which allergens are present or optional. Adult recipes work in smaller servings for toddlers, and when made into purées they are perfect as baby's meals.

Part Three considers some of the research and recommendations around food allergies, and how changes over the past 20 years in the way we live, shop and eat may have contributed to an increase in food allergies. As well, young babies can suffer from many symptoms that mimic allergies and food intolerances. The rise of reflux in children and adults today is concerning, and we give you simple explanations, ways to manage reflux and guidance on when to seek medical advice.

Making decisions on what to feed your family can be challenging, so it is my goal that the practical advice in this book on the common food allergies, as well as serving up real food cooked right to your children from the very beginning, will diminish any fear of food and empower you to raise healthy, adventurous eaters.

I wish you and your family a lifetime journey of fabulous food together.

Follow our story on **www.wecanalleatthat.com**

PAM BROOK

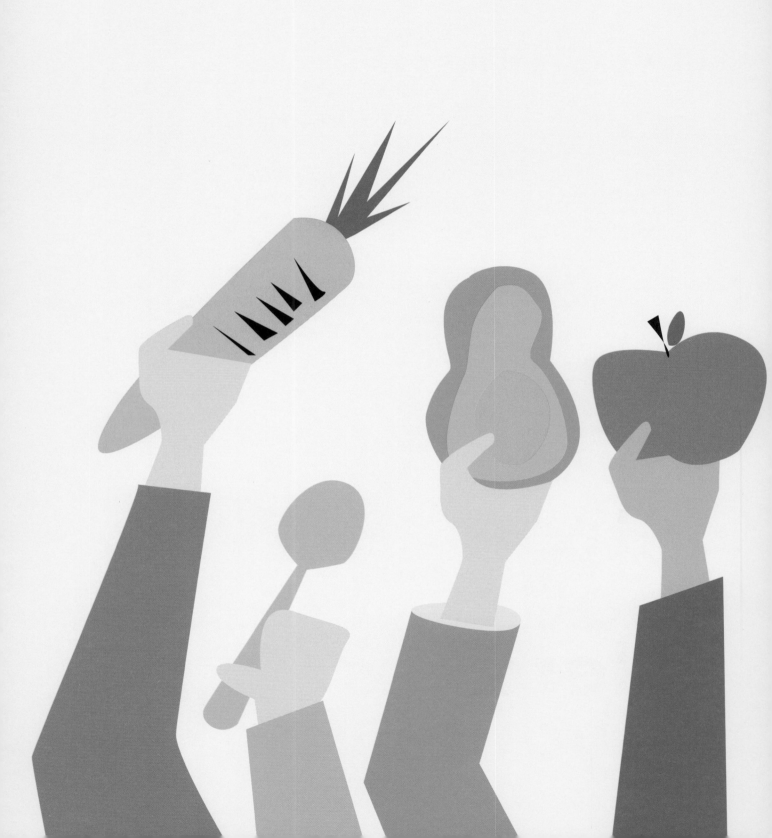

Introducing food and food allergens to your baby

Home cooking creates healthier families

Over the years I've seen many extreme food trends come and go. There's been a dramatic increase in the variety of processed foods available. This increase seemingly offers more choice but has in fact narrowed the range and reduced the nutritional value of the food we are giving to our children.

As a result, there has also been an increasing move away from home cooking. Advertisers and marketers have lured us into believing it's an easier and better choice to buy takeaway or processed food because we're busy. Then in 2020 came the COVID-19 pandemic and many people changed their cooking and eating practices overnight. When people all around the world went into isolation during the pandemic, they started cooking at home because they had to, and discovered that home cooking really can be affordable, fun and delicious.

The benefits of home cooking

There are so many reasons to cook and enjoy food at home with your family - nutritional, financial and social. For starters, families who cook at home tend to eat a healthier diet with more fresh fruit and vegetables and fewer processed and junk foods. But cooking at home isn't just about creating healthier, more nutritious meals. As well as making good food choices, it's about the other benefits that flow when your family cooks and eats together. At my house the family shares meals, conversation and our daily highs and lows around the dinner table. It's a way of life and cooking that inspires me, as well as chefs Sarah Swan and Sam Gowing, every day.

My kids and grandchildren have been around me in the kitchen since they were 6 months old. Children learn about food by sight, touch, taste, feel and smell, and by being part of the preparation process. Children who help to cook experience a range of flavours and are more likely to eat foods they have helped make - or, better yet, grow - and become more adventurous eaters. When children help to cook it can start with the simplest fun things, such as licking the bowl or spoon, passing the vegies or peeling the banana. Forget perfect presentation, forget perfect attention to detail - just make it fun and delicious.

The many reasons why people don't cook - 'no time', 'nothing in the fridge', 'I'm a lousy cook' - can usually be overcome with a little planning. If you're time-poor (and who isn't?), it's a good idea to plan ahead for ingredients. You could even create a meal plan for the week on Sunday and work up a shopping list. Shopping with a purpose means you're likely to only buy what you need, thereby saving money and reducing waste. As well, shopping only for what is in season means you get the highest quality produce at the lowest price.

If you don't have many opportunities to cook, when you do get around to it perhaps cook a large batch and freeze some for later. Make sure you label the container with the contents and date. (See also Storing, refrigerating and freezing on page 31.) You can also find creative ways to cook with leftovers (such as our Bubble and squeak recipe on page 74).

Of course, cooking comes easier to some than others. Some people love cooking, but others may never have been taught the simple how-tos, or are terrified to follow a recipe in case they don't get it exactly right. But practice makes perfect - never surrender is my advice. If you follow the basic recipe steps and practise and persist, you can do it. These days there are also plenty of step-by-step videos available on the internet to help you learn new techniques. It's never too late to learn to cook. Don't aim for perfection, just good food.

Home cooking for children with allergies

Most adults and children are allergy-free and this means having a huge range of choices. However, a small but growing number of both children and adults have food allergies. The good news is that 90 per cent of children don't, and many children who are severely affected in their early years can outgrow it. Most children with cow's milk, wheat, egg or soy allergies will outgrow them (see page 230), but many children who are allergic to shellfish, peanuts and tree nuts will have to manage their allergy for the rest of their lives, or until research finds new treatments and cures. (See Part Three: Understanding food allergies and related conditions.)

If your child has allergies you will need to prepare meals that fit their needs, but these meals can often still work for all the family. It's so much easier when everyone in the house is eating the same meal - one that can be easily adapted for different ages or needs. Most of the recipes in this book are designed to be served to the whole family, with a few tweaks to make them suitable for babies or toddlers.

If your child has allergies it's all the more reason to cook with fresh ingredients at home, so you know where your food comes from as well as everything it contains. In each recipe in this book we have listed all the food allergens and optional food allergens, and we give you many alternatives if you need to exclude an ingredient. Of course there are some great resources, cookbooks and recipes out there, written specifically for people with allergies and/or food intolerances, which I encourage you to look up if you need more help or ideas.[1]

Eating together

Home-cooked family meals and eating together are good for the mind, body and soul. They can make your family feel more connected - more than almost any other activity can. It's not just me saying that. Medical researchers have observed that families who regularly eat home-cooked meals together (five times per week or more) have been found to be happier and healthier and to eat less processed foods, sugar and junk food.[2]

Eating meals together teaches your children that mealtimes are both a family tradition and an essential daily routine. Children of all ages love the connection that happens at family meals. Often everyone's busy doing their own thing during the day, so dinner (or weekend lunch) is a special time when everyone can be together. It helps your children to feel positive about food and eating as a shared experience. What's not at the table is just as important - no screens, mobile phones or tablets. It's family time!

Mealtimes should not be a battleground about food. Avoid giving your children too many snacks before dinner, and be firm but fair, and flexible, about kids finishing everything on their plate - I still have an aversion to overcooked green beans from a time when my mum insisted I eat everything on the plate! Parents need to be the leaders. People say that if the child observes a parent being fussy, they may be fussy too, but none of us are perfect, so just do the best you can.

THE BENEFITS OF FAMILY MEALTIMES

- **Family mealtimes improve your children's mental and physical wellbeing and general health.**

- **Regular mealtimes encourage less snacking.**

- **Your children's communication skills will improve.**

- **Mealtime conversations improve children's vocabulary – children who have a better vocabulary may find reading easier and may learn to read earlier.**

- **Mealtimes improve your children's fine-motor skills and hand-eye coordination.**

- **If the family makes good meal choices, your children will also eat more fruit and vegetables, have a healthier, more balanced diet and consume less junk food, fried foods and soft drinks.**

- **Children are likely to eat more healthily when they grow up and move out of home.**

- **Eating meals together reduces TV and screen hours.**

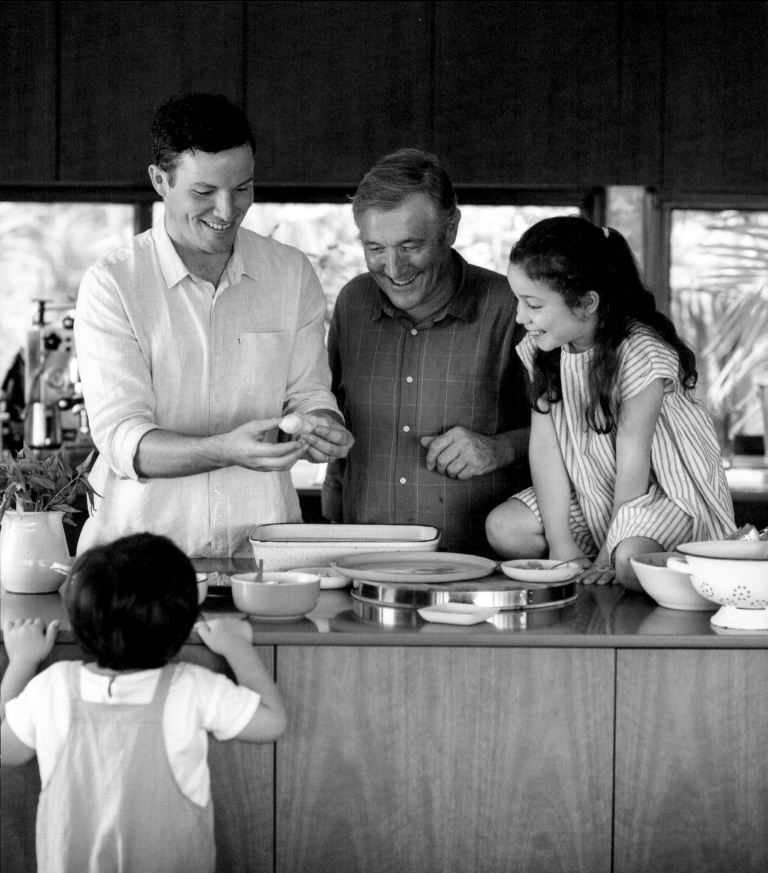

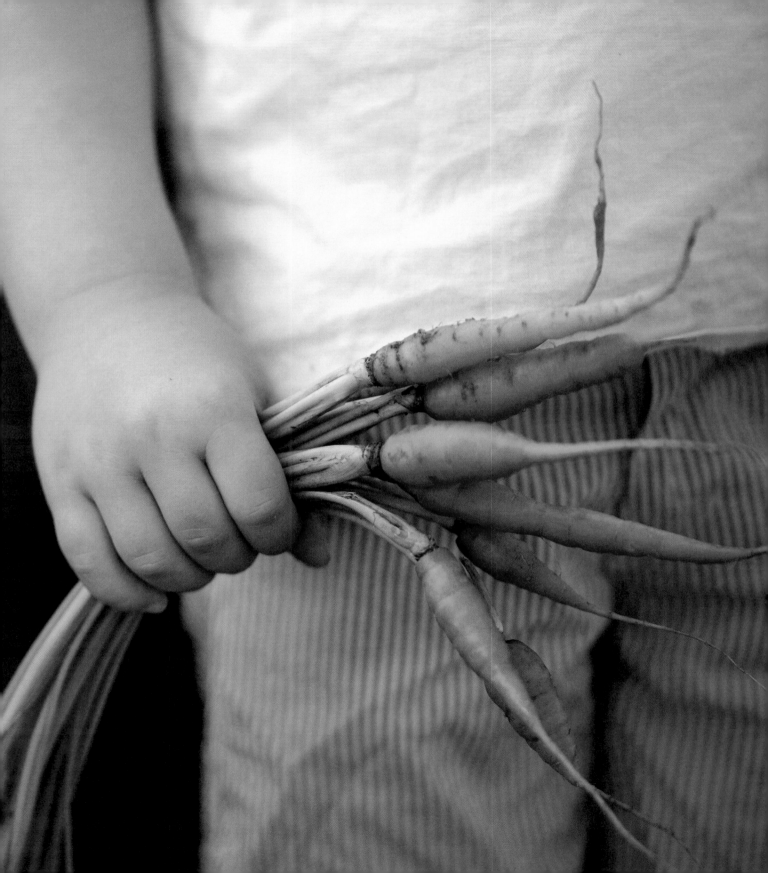

When is my baby ready for solid food?

There are various signs to look out for that will let you know when your baby is ready for solid food. However, generally you can introduce solids at around 6 months of age, but not before 4 months.

Around 6 months (not before 4 months)

Signs your baby is ready for solid food will be an increased appetite, wanting to feed more frequently and looking for more after just drinking breast milk or infant formula. At this stage your baby should be able to sit upright - at the very beginning sitting supported on your lap, and later in a highchair. They will be like a baby sparrow showing interest in the foods you are eating as they start to look around for real food, with their mouth open when a spoon of goodness comes their way. As your baby switches from suckling to learning to eat solid foods, their swallow starts to change from a tongue thrust - where half of everything you feed seems to come back out - to a proper swallow, followed by learning to chew.

Why home-made baby food is best

Fresh food prepared at home, free of additives and preservatives, is the best choice for your baby. Their digestive system is immature and still developing, and it's important to choose first foods that are gentle on their tummy. Much of the baby food eaten today is processed and comes from pouches or packets. Processed food is usually quite acidic and, in fact, has to be acidic by law to prevent bacterial growth. You'll commonly see these foods have added citric acid or ascorbic acid. The most acidic foods are the 'wet' food in pouches and baby food in jars or tins. It's best to save processed foods for when you are 'on the go' and have no other choices and absolutely need the convenience of a packaged food. If your baby suffers from reflux (see page 240), you should be cautious with processed foods, as a diet rich in acidic foods can make reflux worse.[3] Freezing home-made food in convenient, on-the-go storage containers is a much better choice than buying prepared food.

Baby's first family mealtimes

When your baby moves from your lap and can sit in a highchair, they're ready for meals with all the family. They will begin to see mealtimes as a special family experience and they will learn so much by watching what you eat and how you eat it. Make it easy for yourself and be prepared for messy hands, hair and faces when you serve baby's first foods. Bibs and cloths to catch stray food are essential, and perhaps a towel under the highchair to catch what goes over the side.

How to serve baby their first foods

The first time you give baby solid food, choose a moment when they are relaxed and content and just getting hungry. Sometimes the first taste of a new food will be offered on a parent's fingertip. But learning to eat from a spoon is a messy but essential part of your child's development as they learn to enjoy real food like the rest of the family.

Your child can see and smell food on a spoon, and it's part of learning about foods - not just what they taste like but what they look like too. As adults we like to eat food that looks enticing, and it's just the same for baby. **Always stay with your baby while they are eating, as they are learning to develop their swallow and their eating skills.**

How much food to serve baby?

Keep the total amount of food small - the first time 1-2 teaspoons may be plenty, progressing to 1-2 tablespoons of food in total. There should be no rush to replace breast milk or formula with solid foods, so make sure you keep your baby's portion size balanced and don't overfeed - your baby is still learning what a full tummy feels like, and their tummies are much smaller than ours. Your baby will let you know when they've had enough by losing interest in the food or pushing the spoon away.

Start with smooth textures

Serving small amounts of smooth purées that are easy to swallow is the secret to early success. Foods that are too chunky will be difficult to swallow and are a choking risk; foods that are too runny will dribble everywhere; smooth purées will be just right. (For more information on preparing and puréeing baby's food, see Best cooking methods on page 29.)

Many of your baby's tastebuds are on the roof of their mouth, and how the texture of their food feels when their tongue presses it against the roof of their mouth often decides whether they accept or reject it. Your baby learns how to handle different food textures with experience, from fluid drinks through to slippery textures such as yoghurt, as well as smooth and grainy textures and thick purées - likewise they will learn about cold and warm temperatures. However, it's your responsibility to ensure you don't serve hot food to baby.

Allow time for digestion

Try not to lay your baby down straight after eating, so their little tummies have time to digest food while they are in the upright position. It's best to feed your child their solids a few hours before bedtime so they have time to move around, play with family or take their evening bath and digest their food before lying down to sleep.

Baby-led weaning

An alternative way of starting baby's first foods is by baby-led weaning.[4] This method means you forget about purées and spoon-feeding; instead, when your baby can grasp foods well, usually between 6 and 8 months, you give them nutritious but soft finger foods. For baby-led weaning, texture is everything. Finger foods should be soft and easy to smash with gentle pressure between your thumb and finger, and fruits and vegetables should be steamed to soften them. Meats and seafood should be moist and shredded into tiny strips or pieces. The idea of baby-led weaning is to give babies a chance to explore foods themselves, but it does rely on their development of grasping and holding foods. Baby-led weaning is naturally more messy than spoon-feeding, as the path from hand to mouth takes time in the beginning. Make sure you give your child time and nutritional balance with the mix of foods you prepare. If you can't get the dietary balance right, don't be afraid to mix baby-led weaning with some puréed spoon-fed meals. **You will need to closely supervise your child as they eat to prevent choking.**

Developing baby's love of flavours, textures and aromas

Whether you spoon-feed or try baby-led weaning, keep your baby's diet varied and let them experience increasingly lumpy and challenging textures as they become ready, as well as new flavours.

Your baby's diet should start simply, then gradually embrace a variety of different flavours and textures over time. It's best to try new foods when baby is hungry rather than at the end of a meal. In this book we keep it simple to start with, using single-ingredient purées (see page 29), gradually progressing to adapted versions of recipes designed for the whole family, which will provide a fabulous exploration of flavours.

Give your baby time to appreciate new flavours and don't rush it. Don't ever force a food on your child - meals need to be a pleasurable time. Your baby will also enjoy playing with their food and feeling different textures - get the camera out!

Food preferences are largely learnt and, although a child may push a spoon with a new food away, the research shows that it may take up to eight attempts before a child will finally accept or reject a new food. Don't force it - be creative, persistent and patient. If your baby truly doesn't like it, maybe try again in a few months.

Sometimes you might want to present the same food in different ways. For example, with baby's first vegetable purée, try adding a dollop of it to yoghurt instead of serving it on its own, or mix it with another purée, or you might roast the vegies instead of steaming to create naturally caramelised flavours. (This is great for slightly bitter foods such as cauliflower and broccoli.)

ALWAYS TASTE BABY'S FOOD YOURSELF

We recommend you taste your child's food before you feed them. This doesn't mean season it to your taste, but try the food so you understand the textures and flavours your baby likes.

Baby's tastebuds and digestive system are immature, and they are more sensitive to strong flavours. However, that doesn't mean we shouldn't create flavourful meals for them. Start simple and, over the next months and years, they will gradually come to enjoy and share more strongly flavoured foods like the rest of the family. In the recipe section in Part Two you will see that for babies we recommend leaving out, or reducing, some strongly flavoured or overly salty ingredients, but these can be slowly introduced when your child hits the toddler age of 1–3 years. Of course, some children will naturally be more adventurous eaters than others.

The smell of most foods is learnt from an early age, with the possible exception of 'off' or decayed foods. Children's food preferences are very much influenced by the aromas and flavours that are common in the house and by the attitudes of family and friends.

Sweet, salty and bitter flavours

You can help guide your children in the tastes that they grow up with. Most children have a tendency towards sweet before the age of 12 months, but if you give your child predominantly sweet foods they will develop a sweet tooth and may reject flavours that aren't sweet. If you keep their diet varied you will create more adventurous eaters. Babies tend to develop a preference for naturally salty flavours after 4 months of age. However, in babies under 12 months their kidneys can only cope with a small amount of salt - less than 1 gram per day (⅕ teaspoon). Therefore, you should limit salty foods and sauces. (See Salt on page 42.)

Babies - like many adults! - have a natural liking of foods with a slightly fatty mouthfeel, so adding a touch of fat to foods can lift their flavour appeal. For example, add ⅛ teaspoon ghee or butter to mashed vegetables or puréed bitter greens. (See Fats on page 43.) Small amounts of bitter flavours, such as English spinach, broccoli and cauliflower, are good to introduce early to help your baby develop an acceptance and appreciation of bitter tastes. Subtly adding slightly bitter foods to naturally sweeter or richer foods helps baby develop a taste for foods of many and varied flavours. Adding a balancing touch of sour/acid, using lime or lemon in appropriate recipes, helps develop your baby's flavour palate.

SERVE MORE VEGETABLES THAN FRUIT

It's important to feed your baby more vegies than fruit so their diet is healthy, diverse and not overly sweet. Carrot, potato, parsnip, leek, carrot, zucchini (courgette), baby squash and swede (rutabaga) are delicious introductions to vegies.

First fruits should be easy for your baby to digest - preferably ripe fruits that are not too tart, such as pears, red-skinned apples, bananas and melon. Fruits are naturally sweeter than vegetables, so if these dominate your child's first foods, your child will tend to always look for sweeter meals.

Drinks

For the first 12 months your child will be breastfed, or on infant formula. On hot days and between meals, water is the best drink. Developing a taste for water - rather than juice or sugary drinks - is a crucial part of your baby's taste development. Fruit juices are a concentrated source of fruit sugars and should always be diluted - ideally a ratio of 1:4 juice to water. Your baby should have no more than one glass per day.

Sweet, sugary soft drinks are highly acidic to babies' and toddlers' tummies, and the average can of soft drink may contain up to 10 teaspoons of sugar. If there are no soft drinks in your house, you can't drink them. In my house soft drinks belong in one place - down the drain!

Introducing milk in a cup as an occasional drink is OK, but it's not a meal in itself. It's not appropriate to substitute milk for formula or breast milk before 12 months of age.

KEEP UP THE BREAST MILK AND FORMULA

When you introduce your child to solids it's important to continue breastfeeding or giving their infant formula, which is their main source of nutrition, for the first 12 months. As your child grows and gets much more of their nutrition from solid foods, they will naturally want less breast milk or formula.

Spoons

When your baby becomes interested in a spoon, give them a soft one to play with at mealtimes, from as early as 6 months. Even if they miss all the food, they're slowly learning how to grasp it, drop it, pick it up and generally manage it, while you keep one to actually feed them with. Getting spoon to mouth is a suspenseful journey - food usually finds eyebrows, nose and cheeks before it makes it to the mouth, but the learning is one of those key steps in hand-eye coordination and skill development.

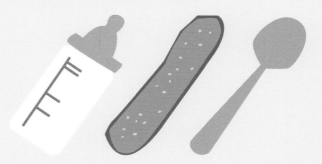

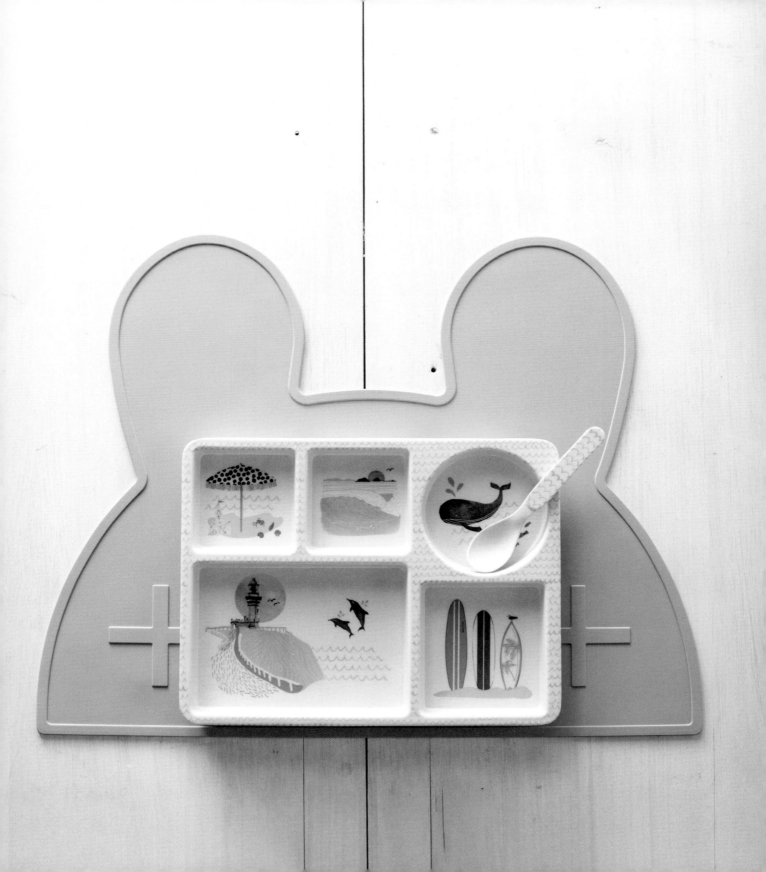

9 months

At 9 months your older baby is ready for soft mushy chunks and lumpy foods, such as mashed banana and pumpkin (squash). You'll need to supervise your child while giving them any chunky foods, but encouraging them with texture is really important in the development of more adventurous eating.

Starting on finger foods

Finger foods are great fun for older babies and toddlers. The average age for introducing finger foods to babies is between 7 and 8 months. Make sure finger foods are soft enough so there is no choking risk, and always supervise your baby while they're eating. Keep the pieces big enough to grip with tiny fingers but soft enough to mush with fingers, gums and first front teeth. Try pieces of soft fruit, such as pear, banana, mango and avocado, or cooked vegies, such as steamed carrot and pumpkin (squash).

Eating safely

Young children may not chew their food well or they may get distracted while eating and try to swallow it whole, making choking a common hazard for children up to the age of 5 years. Round or hard foods are the most dangerous, so be careful with nuts, grapes, popcorn etc. Time spent preparing, chopping or cooking to soften is important early on, and supervision is just as important. For between-meal snacks make sure they're sitting still, and for main meals there is no better place to focus on food than eating with the family.

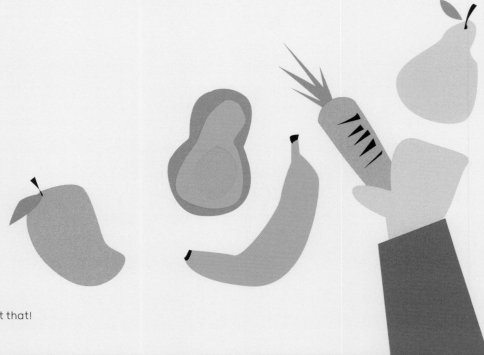

12 months plus

From 12 months your toddler is getting much better with finger foods and is definitely more independent at the dinner table. If you haven't had a chance to let your child experience textures and flavours before this age, then just go at the rate your child prefers. The important thing is to create interesting food with a broad range of flavours early on, so that the variety of foods your child enjoys becomes fully developed. Your toddler will soon be eating smaller serves of the same food the rest of the family is eating, but make sure it is well chopped up into small pieces of about 1 cm (½ in) and that any nuts are finely chopped.

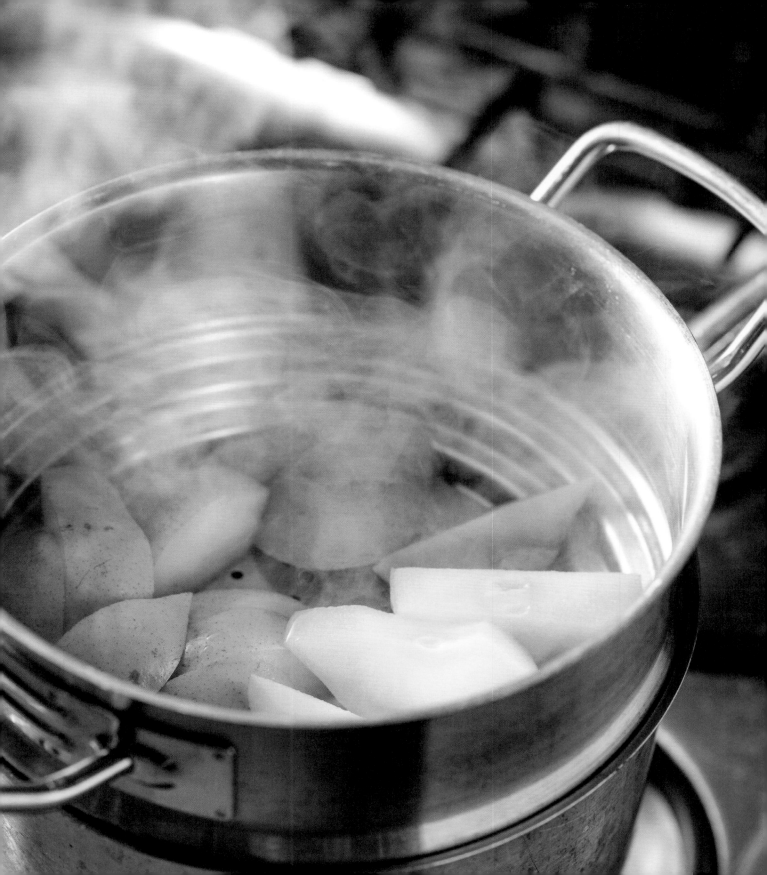

Baby's first foods – the 'cotton wool' weeks

If this is your first baby, during the first few weeks when you move from exclusively breast milk or formula to introducing simple solid food, you may be nervously watching your baby's every mouthful. However, if this is your second or third child you'll probably be feeling much more comfortable. You should keep foods simple for the first few weeks, then try to gradually introduce variety in flavour, aroma, colour and texture (see page 23).

Best cooking methods

For baby's very first foods, start with single-ingredient purées - preferably vegetables rather than fruits to avoid your baby developing a preference for sweet foods. Steaming is the best way to cook foods to preserve vitamins, minerals and nutrition, before puréeing the food to a smooth texture. Always allow the food to cool before serving.

The unpuréed steamed vegies can also work as a side dish for older children and adults, or add steamed fruits to ice cream or yoghurt for dessert - perhaps topped with a crumble-like nut and seed sprinkle. Steamed vegetables are also perfect for older babies and toddlers to enjoy as finger food or as a more lumpy mash.

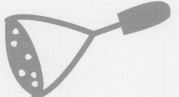

IDEAL FIRST VEGETABLES TO PURÉE

- **Sweet potato**
- **Pumpkin (squash)**
- **Carrot**
- **Parsnip**
- **Potato**
- **Zucchini (courgette) or baby squash**
- **Leek**
- **Swede (rutabaga)**

IDEAL FIRST FRUITS TO PURÉE

Choose ripe, fresh, soft fruits, which can be puréed or mashed finely. Firmer fruits will need to be cooked to soften them before puréeing.

Soft fruits

- **Banana**
- **Papaya**
- **Melon**
- **Avocado (very high in fats so keep amounts small)**

Firmer fruits

- **Apple (red-skinned)**
- **Pear**
- **Stone fruits**

Steaming

Steaming preserves the nutrients in vegetables and fruits more than any other cooking method. Avoid overcooking to preserve as much nutrition, colour and flavour as possible.

If you're using conventionally grown produce, it's important to thoroughly wash off any pesticide residue. If you're using organic produce you still need to wash off any dirt. Rinse in cold water, brush any thick-skinned vegetables and pat them dry with paper towel or a clean tea towel (dish towel). Trim and peel as desired. The smaller the pieces, the faster they will cook.

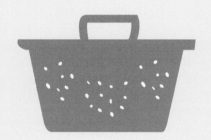

Steaming vegetables in a saucepan

- You will need a small stainless-steel steamer.

- Place the steaming basket in a small- to medium-sized saucepan with the correct lid to fit.

- Pour in enough water to come just below the base of the steamer. Add the vegetables to the steamer. Bring to the boil, reduce the heat and cook as per the table below. When cooked, the vegies should still be full of colour but should be able to be easily pierced with a knife or fork.

- Once cooked, transfer to a colander and cool under cold water. Let the steam evaporate away from your hands and face. Keep drained vegetables warm and use as required. Add a squeeze of lemon and/or a dash of olive oil to preserve colour if you will be using it later.

VEGETABLE STEAMING TIMES

VEGETABLE	STEAMING TIME ON A STOVETOP
Asparagus	3-5 minutes, spears and short pieces
Broccoli	3-5 minutes, stalks and florets
Carrots	7-10 minutes, depending on size
Cauliflower	5-10 minutes, florets
Corn cob portions	7-10 minutes
English spinach	2-3 minutes
Green beans	3-5 minutes, trimmed, depending on size
Peas	3-5 minutes fresh, podded; a little longer for frozen
Potatoes, sliced	7-10 minutes, sliced, depending on size
Silverbeet (Swiss chard)	3-5 minutes, chopped

Steaming fruit

Fresh, soft fruits such as mangoes, ripe bananas and melons can be puréed without steaming. For hard or firm fruits, wash them thoroughly (no need to peel, as the skin contains lots of goodness), cut into bite-sized pieces, then steam until it can be easily pierced with a knife - about 3-5 minutes.

FRUIT STEAMING TIMES

FRUIT	STEAMING TIME ON A STOVETOP
Apples (red-skinned)	3-5 minutes, pips removed, cut into bite-sized pieces
Pears	3-5 minutes, pips removed, cut into bite-sized pieces
Stone fruits • Nectarines • Peaches • Plums	3-5 minutes, stones removed, cut into bite-sized pieces

Cooking vegetables and fruit in a microwave

- Place the vegetables or fruit in a microwave-safe bowl and add a splash of water.

- Cover loosely with a lid or plastic wrap, leaving a small air vent, then microwave on high (100%) for 3-4 minutes, depending on microwave strength. Remove the cover carefully.

- Allow to cool before puréeing and always check that the food isn't too hot for your baby before serving.

Puréeing

For baby's first foods, after steaming you will need to purée them until they are silky smooth with no lumps. Simply add the steamed fruit or vegetable to a food processor or jug blender and blend - or use a hand-held blender. If it's too thick, add a small amount of cooking liquid, breast milk or formula to thin to a silky smooth purée.

Storing, refrigerating and freezing

- Always store food in airtight containers.

- Home-made purées can be stored in sealed containers for up to 2 days in the refrigerator.

- Do not save or store partially eaten foods.

- Freeze extra amounts in small containers, or you can use flexible ice-cube trays stored inside an airtight freezer bag.

- Store frozen foods for a maximum of 3 months.

- Always label containers with the contents and date before freezing.

- Don't refreeze foods that have been previously frozen and thawed.

- You can heat from frozen in a microwave or on the stovetop until fully heated and allow to cool before serving.

- Once food has defrosted, use it within 24 hours.

First foods (the 'cotton wool weeks') meal plans

When your baby first starts on solids, your meal plan for the first week will look something like this:

Week one

Early morning	Breakfast	Lunch	Evening	Bedtime
breast/formula bottle on demand	breast/formula bottle on demand	puréed vegies or fruits breast/formula bottle on demand	breast/formula bottle on demand	breast/formula bottle on demand

As your baby grows and looks for more food after breast or bottle feeding, then add in solids at breakfast.

Week two

Early morning	Breakfast	Lunch	Evening	Bedtime
breast/formula bottle on demand	puréed vegies or fruits – you can add to their first cereal breast/formula bottle on demand	puréed vegies or fruits breast/formula bottle on demand	breast/formula bottle on demand	breast/formula bottle on demand

The last meal to add is dinner. Be aware of not giving too much food in the evening so your baby doesn't go to sleep with a very full tummy. (See Allow time for digestion on page 22.)

Week three

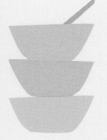

Early morning	Breakfast	Lunch	Evening	Bedtime
breast/formula bottle on demand	puréed vegies or fruits, or first cereal with vegies or fruit breast/formula bottle on demand	add a cooked protein, such as beans, chicken or beef, puréed with vegies breast/formula bottle on demand	puréed mixed vegies or mixed fruits breast/formula bottle on demand	breast/formula bottle on demand

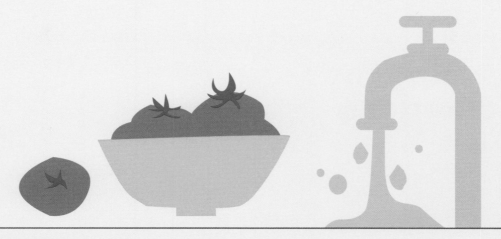

HYGIENE TIPS

Use safe food-handling practices when preparing your baby's meals:

- **Wash your hands thoroughly before preparing meals.**

- **Rinse fresh fruits and vegetables well under running tap water, especially if they are to be served uncooked.**

- **Keep raw meats, poultry, fish and seafood away from cooked food, fresh fruits and vegetables.**

- **Use separate chopping boards for raw meat, fish and vegetables.**

- **Store cooked foods appropriately in the refrigerator or freezer (for more information see page 31).**

- **Discard any leftovers from baby's plate.**

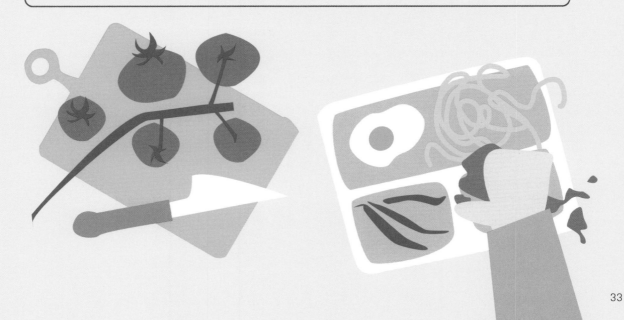

When and why to start introducing the common food allergens

The common food allergens are foods that commonly cause food allergies.

Allergy experts around the world, including the British Society for Allergy & Clinical Immunology, the Australasian Society of Clinical Immunology and Allergy, and the American Academy of Allergy, Asthma and Immunology, now advise that early introduction of the common food allergens to children between the ages of 6 and 12 months may greatly reduce the risk of them developing an allergy to those foods. Studies of babies at high risk of having allergies have shown that this reduces the chance of them developing food allergies.[6] See page 229 for other factors that may reduce the risk of developing allergies.

In this age of 'free from' foods, which surround us on supermarket shelves, it's easy for many families to unintentionally never introduce the common food allergens to their baby. The recommendation of allergy experts is that once your baby is used to their early solid foods, such as a range of vegetable and fruit purées and proteins, then you should carefully start introducing the common food allergens. Once successfully introduced, you should continue to make these foods part of your child's regular diet.

How to introduce the common food allergens to your baby

Just like you, your baby needs variety in food for a balanced diet. This helps develop their palate as they experience different tastes and flavours. The introduction of common food allergens to your baby's diet follows the same philosophy and requires just a little patience, but will build your confidence in creating delicious recipes.

When introducing the common food allergens, start with just one at a time. If you are concerned your child may have food allergies, you can choose a more cautious approach and rub a small amount of the food inside your baby's lip to start with. If there is no allergic reaction after a few minutes, start serving a small amount of the allergen, say ¼ teaspoon mixed into your child's food. Keep a watch over them for the next 30 minutes. If your child does have an allergic reaction it will usually occur fairly quickly after eating - stop feeding that food and seek medical advice from your doctor or allergist. (For more information on allergic reactions see page 225.)

If you are more confident, then the first time you can simply add a small amount to your baby's puréed food.

Don't test new foods by rubbing them on baby's skin. Some foods may stain or irritate the skin and cause minor redness around the mouth, which doesn't necessarily mean that there is a food allergy. When redness has occurred, gently clean your baby's face with a soft, moist cloth, then monitor them as detailed opposite. (See Skin sensitivity versus allergic reaction on page 226.)

Once you are sure your baby tolerates the first food allergen, you can start to add the next one. Allow for any delayed reactions before introducing a new food allergen, but go at the pace that suits you and your baby. How quickly you progress depends on your child and any history of allergies and intolerances. For a child with no allergic history, we recommend waiting 2-3 days between the introduction of each food allergen. If you are unsure, always seek your doctor's or paediatric allergist's advice.

After the first month or two of solids, or when you are confident your baby is tolerating and enjoying all the foods and common food allergens you've given them so far, you can start to introduce more complex recipes that all the family can enjoy together (with obvious adaptations to suit your baby's age). See the recipes in Part Two of this book.

For more information see Part Three: Understanding food allergies and related conditions.

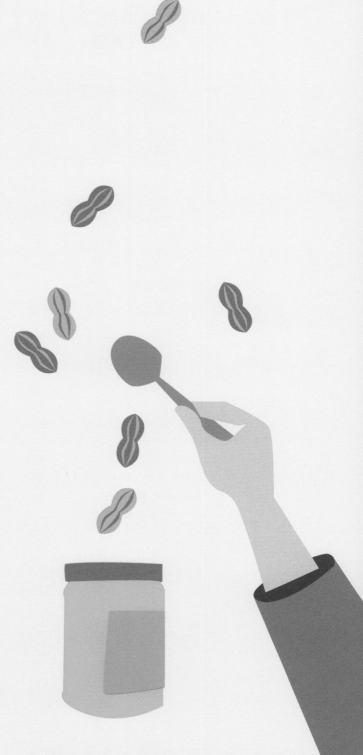

The common food allergens

The most common food allergens today are peanut, tree nut, dairy, egg, sesame, and fish and shellfish. Allergies to soy and wheat are slightly less common. Here we discuss the common food allergens and ways to introduce them into your baby's diet. There are many other foods children can be allergic to, but we've focused on the most common ones. (See also Other food allergens on the rise on page 230.)

Some foods have a cross-allergenicity with other foods because they contain similar proteins. For example, people with peanut allergies are also likely to be allergic to lupins and vice versa. Where there is a common cross-allergenicity we've noted it.

Nuts

All nuts are not the same. Peanuts are actually legumes, not nuts, and are sometimes called groundnuts. Children with allergies to peanuts are not necessarily allergic to tree nuts and vice versa.

When introducing your baby to nuts it's important to make sure the nuts are in the form of a flour/meal or in a smooth butter/paste with no crunchy or lumpy pieces. Start with the smallest amount of nut butter (⅛ - ¼ teaspoon) on your fingertip for your child to suck on, or it can be mixed into your baby's meals. You can buy nut butters in your supermarket (check the ingredients carefully for any other allergens to make sure it is a pure nut butter, and always choose smooth pastes with no added sugar or salt) or make them at home in a food processor (see Home-made nut butters on page 217).

A touch of fat, such as from nuts, adds flavour, and babies love slightly fatty foods (see Fats on page 43). An easy way to introduce nuts regularly to your baby's food is to add a small amount of a nut butter or unrefined nut oil to a dish.

PEANUTS

You can introduce peanuts by adding just a small amount of smooth, unsalted peanut butter to your baby's meal - say about ⅛-¼ teaspoon.

CROSS-ALLERGENICITY: Peanuts come from the same legume family as lupins, so an allergy to peanuts can mean your child will also be allergic to lupins (found in a wide range of food products).

TREE NUTS

The tree nuts that are most important to introduce are the ones your child may have the most contact with in your home; in your family's, friends' or carers' homes; and in the external environment. (See Sensitisation and developing oral tolerance on page 236.)

Tree nuts include:

- Almond
- Macadamia nut
- Pecan
- Walnut
- Hazelnut
- Cashew nut
- Pistachio nut
- Brazil nut
- Pine nut

Easy tree nut butters to make at home are macadamia, cashew and hazelnut. Using nuts without skins, such as blanched almonds or hazelnuts, makes a more liquid paste. Almonds, pecans and walnuts are much drier, so you may need to add a little matching nut oil or a cold-pressed or expeller-pressed oil, such as sunflower or rice-bran oil, to get a smooth paste. Walnuts and pecans are strong-tasting nuts and we recommend you blend these nuts with other flavours that balance the bitterness, such as a carrot or pear purée.

CROSS-ALLERGENICITY: Walnuts and pecans come from the same family, so an allergy to pecans can mean your child will also be allergic to walnuts. Likewise, cashew nuts and pistachio nuts come from the same tree-nut family, so an allergy to cashew nuts can mean your child will also be allergic to pistachio nuts.

Dairy

A dairy allergy is very different from lactose intolerance. Lactose intolerance is the inability of your baby's digestive system to digest lactose, which is the sugar found in cow's, goat's and sheep's milk. In a dairy allergy, the immune system identifies the proteins in milk, such as whey protein and casein, as a threat and creates an allergic reaction. Cow's milk allergies currently affect up to 3 per cent of children.

Dairy foods include:

- Full-cream (whole) cow's or goat's milk
- Cream
- Full-fat yoghurt
- Cheese - e.g. soft fresh cheeses, such as ricotta or cottage cheese, or mild cheeses such as cheddar
- Hard cheeses, such as parmesan, pecorino and vintage cheddars, should be used in moderation for younger babies

Small amounts of milk or cream can be mixed with your baby's meals, such as baby cereal or vegetable purée. Yoghurt is more concentrated in casein, so keep introductory amounts small and add it to puréed vegetables or fruits. Yoghurt has the added benefit of its natural probiotic content for gut health (see Probiotics on page 42). Greek yoghurt is simply regular yoghurt that has been strained to make a thicker, richer yoghurt.

CROSS-ALLERGENICITY: If your child has an allergy to cow's milk, they will most likely be allergic to goat's and sheep's milk, and vice versa.

Eggs

It's important to make sure eggs, or foods you make containing eggs, are thoroughly cooked for your baby. The eggs can be scrambled, poached or hard-boiled, or be an ingredient in a cake or slice, but they need to be cooked through. This ensures any bacteria in the egg is killed in the cooking process.

Paediatricians advise not to give babies under 12 months raw egg yolk because of the low but possible risk of salmonella infection. You can introduce egg by adding just a small amount of cooked egg to your baby's meal.

CROSS-ALLERGENICITY: If your child has an allergy to chicken eggs, they will most likely be allergic to duck eggs, and vice versa.

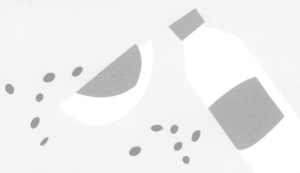

Sesame

The ideal way to introduce sesame is with store-bought tahini paste - or make your own by blending sesame seeds to a paste in your food processor. (White or black sesame seeds are both fine.) You can also use a store-bought hummus that contains tahini, or better still make your own (see our recipe on page 198). Sesame oil is a strong flavour so use just a small amount in cooking.

Sources of sesame include:

- Tahini - check the ingredients list for any other allergens
- Mild hummus containing tahini - avoid strongly spiced hummus
- Sesame oil

Soy

For babies under 12 months omit condiments such as soy sauce and miso because of their high salt content. For toddlers and adults we recommend using a naturally fermented soy sauce or a tamari free from additives and preservatives (see Salt on page 42).

Sources of soy include:

- **Fresh soy beans (edamame) - easy to add to vegetable purées**
- **Tofu (silken or firm)**
- **Soy milk**

Fish and shellfish

Fish and shellfish have quite different flavours compared to fruits and vegetables so, as a flavour experience and an allergen introduction, start your baby with just small amounts added to their other foods as part of a meal.

FISH

Avoid the larger fish that are higher up the food chain, such as shark, tuna, marlin and swordfish - they tend to contain more heavy metals, such as mercury - and instead choose the smaller fish. It's ideal to start with a soft white fish, such as snapper, cod or jewfish, and then progress to the stronger-flavoured, oilier, omega-3-rich fish, such as salmon and trout. **Make sure you carefully remove all bones from the fish, as these are a choking hazard!**

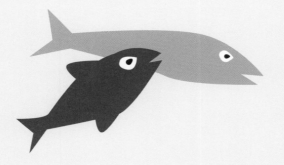

SHELLFISH

With shellfish, start with just a small amount that's easy to purée and add it to other foods, such as potato, pasta and vegetable purées. Choose the shellfish your family most commonly eats - needless to say, lobster is not that common in the average household!

Shellfish includes:

- **Prawns (shrimp)**
- **Scallops**
- **Pipis and clams (vongole)**
- **Crab**
- **Lobster and crayfish**

Wheat

One of the main sources of wheat is flour and it can be found in so many foods, such as bread and other baked goods, pasta and noodles. Choose breads that are low in sodium and salt, preferably baked fresh with no preservatives or additives. Sourdough bread is naturally fermented and a delicious choice.

Wheat can be found in:

- **Plain (all-purpose) and wholegrain flour**
- **Quality durum wheat pasta and noodles**
- **Wheatgerm**
- **Wheat bran**
- **Soy sauce** (made with fermented soy beans and wheat; tamari is a good substitute if you need something gluten free, but always check the label)

LESS COMMON FOOD ALLERGENS

- Kiwifruit
- Lupin (which has cross-allergenicity with peanuts)
- Buckwheat - more common in Japan and Korea
- Mustard - more common in Europe, Canada and India
- Celery - more common in Europe

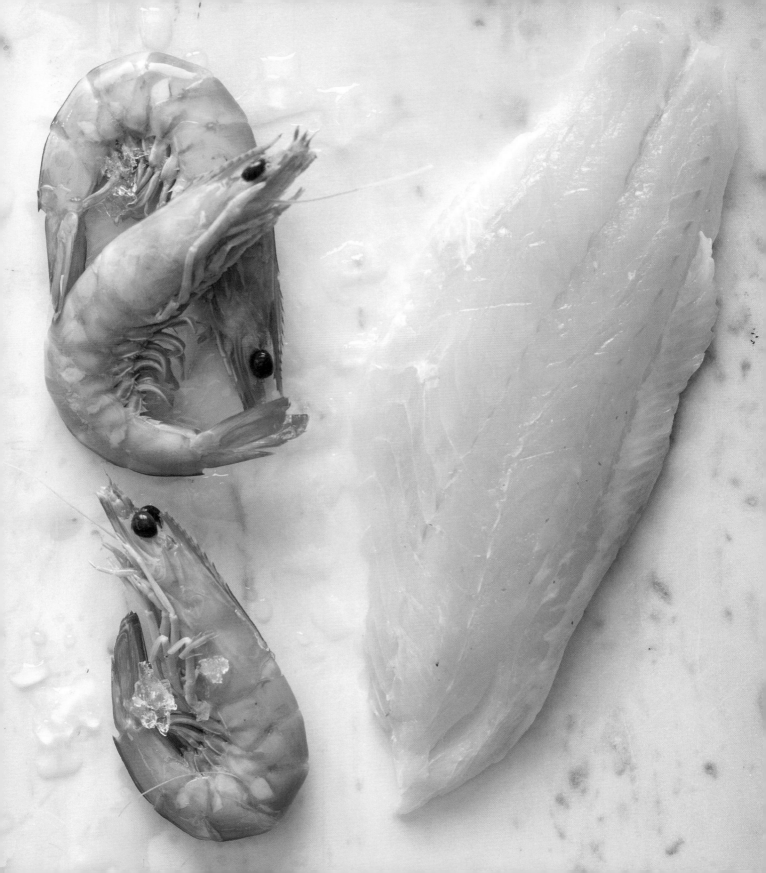

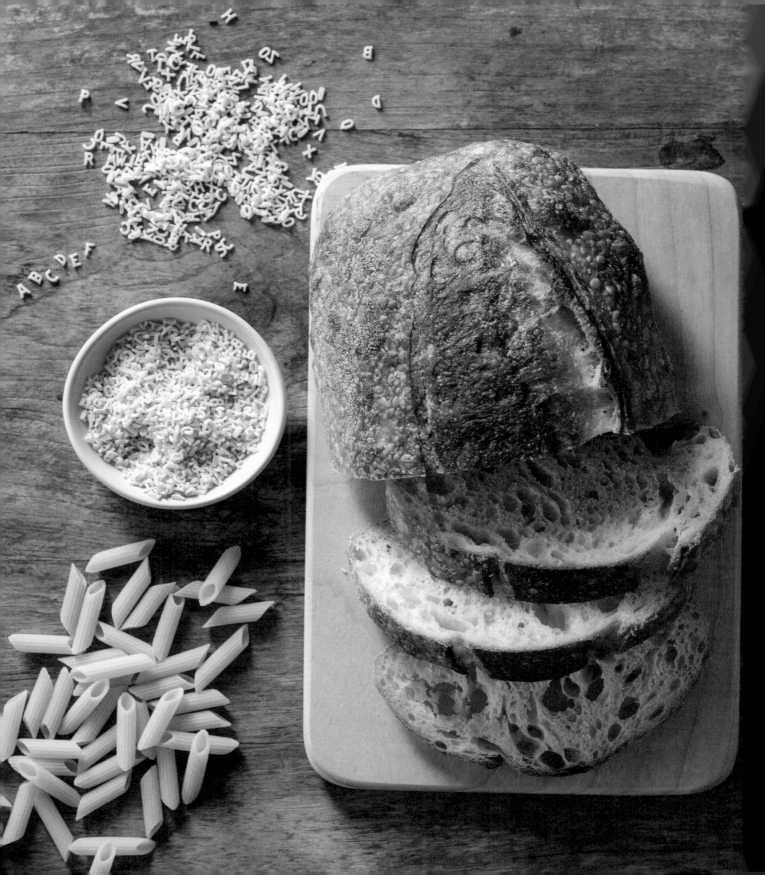

Nutritional basics

It's important that you, your baby and all your family eat a balanced, healthy diet.

Cooking with fresh produce, preferably in-season and organic, gives your family the best start. 'Eat food, not too much, mostly plants' is the famous line by Michael Pollan[7] and steers us in the right direction for choosing what we eat. Following are a few guidelines regarding the major food groups and nutrients.

Vegetables and fruit

Eat more vegetables than fruit. Choose foods that cover the full colour range from red, yellow and green, to white, purple and even blue. Vegetables are often the neglected food in our diet, as fruits are sweeter, ready to go and easier to prepare. Vegetables are rich sources of iron and minerals and essential for good nutrition, so always check that they are the major part of every meal. Adding vegetables also creates meals of greater variety and flavour for the whole family. Fruits are a great source of vitamins, minerals and dietary fibre.

Protein

Protein is an essential part of a healthy diet. Your baby needs enough protein for about 15 per cent of their daily energy/calorie needs. Choose protein from natural food sources, such as meat, fish and seafood, eggs and dairy, and plant protein sources, such as non-GMO soy products, legumes (beans, peas and lentils), nuts and seeds.

Carbohydrates

Carbohydrates are an important source of fuel for our bodies. But it's important to eat carbohydrates from healthy foods, such as whole grains, fruits and vegetables, which are rich in vitamins, minerals and fibre, and avoid carbohydrate-rich processed foods, such as junk foods, white bread and soft drinks.

Fibre

A balanced diet with whole grains, fruits and vegetables provides fibre and helps you and your baby develop a healthy gut microbiome. Your child's microbiome is made up of a huge variety of microbes including bacteria, fungi and viruses, which live inside the intestines. A healthy gut microbiome is essential for good digestion and healthy metabolism, and plays an important role in the development of the immune system. (See also Probiotics on page 42.)

The dietary fibre in your child's food helps develop their microbiome. The less fibre they eat, the less diverse their gut bacteria. Some of the most fibre-rich foods for toddlers are:

- **WHOLEGRAIN BREADS AND CEREALS**
- **VEGETABLES** such as carrots, parsnips, peas, broccoli, kale, beetroot (beets) and beetroot greens and cabbage, to name a few
- **FRESH FRUIT** such as apples, pears, oranges, bananas, berries and prunes
- **LEGUMES** such as dried beans, split peas and lentils
- **NUTS AND SEEDS** such as tree nuts, peanuts, chia seeds and linseeds (flax seeds)

When science first discovered bacteria, all of them were thought to be bad. However, now we know that there are also 'good' bacteria, and we need all the healthy combinations of them that live inside us and on the food we grow. Scientific research into what makes up a healthy microbiome in both children and adults is an important focus in modern medical research today.[8]

Bacteria that are helpful for your gut health are called probiotics, and some that occur naturally in fermented foods can be beneficial. Keep it simple by getting your probiotics from natural food sources. Yoghurt and kefir are usually dairy-based fermented foods naturally containing the beneficial probiotic *Lactobacillus*. These can also be made from soy or coconut milk.

Some fermented foods are not suitable for babies as they are salty, and should be used cautiously. Miso, for example, is quite high in salt so use it sparingly and only for children over 12 months of age.

Salt

Babies need only a small amount of salt - less than 1 gram (⅛ teaspoon) per day - until they are 12 months old. Much of this is found naturally in foods, so when you are adding salt to your meals, do so after putting your baby's serve aside. For adults use just enough salt to balance the flavour in home-cooked meals. Avoid high-salt, processed foods and avoid seasoning your child's food with salty sauces and pastes.

Why do some recipes need salt?

There are certain cooking processes for babies where it's OK to add salt, as the salt helps the cooking process and is drained off before serving - such as adding salt to boiling water to cook pasta and vegetables.

Sugar

Too much sugar can cause tooth decay, and excess sugary foods, which are high in calories, can make you and your baby overweight. Naturally occurring sugars in fruits, vegetables and milk are healthy sugars. Dried fruits have more concentrated fruit sugars, so moderation is important. Avoid sugary processed foods, soft drink, confectionery, cookies and snacks - if they're not in the house you won't eat them, nor will your baby or children, and you'll feel better for it. Limit added sugars, such as regular sugar, maple syrup and agave. Try to only use these in recipes that use added sugar as an essential ingredient. (Paediatricians recommend avoiding honey until after 12 months of age as it may contain spores of bacteria that can cause botulism.)

Why do some recipes need sugar?

Cooked sugars are sticky and it's this stickiness that binds ingredients together. If you remove sugar from a baked recipe, for example muffins or cakes, you will eliminate the sticky component and usually end up with a crumbly end product. So, in this case it's necessary to use sugar.

Essential vitamins and minerals

You and your baby need a balanced, wholefood diet to provide the full range of necessary vitamins and minerals. We've listed just a few good sources below as a starting point.

- **CALCIUM:** dairy, tofu, soy beans, nuts
- **IRON:** legumes, liver, red meat, dark green leafy vegetables, such as English spinach and kale
- **IODINE:** seafood, wholegrain breads, seaweed, dairy products, eggs
- **ZINC:** meat, seafood, legumes, nuts and seeds, dairy, eggs, whole grains
- **VITAMIN C:** citrus fruit, berries, broccoli, potatoes
- **VITAMIN A:** carrots, sweet potatoes
- **VITAMIN B:** fish, meats (liver is great), chicken, grains, legumes, leafy greens
- **VITAMIN D:** sardines, salmon – and sunshine (see The sunshine vitamin on page 235)
- **VITAMIN E:** nuts and seeds, nut and seed oils (preferably cold-pressed or expeller-pressed)

Fats

Babies like slightly fatty foods. Fats add to our experience of food by creating a special 'mouthfeel' or smoothness, plus they help dissolve flavours and seasonings and spread flavours through the food. Fats makes us feel fuller longer and slow down digestion. This is why we feel full after eating dairy, nuts and avocados.

Fats are one of the most misunderstood areas of a baby's nutrition and families are often confused by what are 'good' and 'bad' fats. Here is a list of the most commonly known fats:

- **MONOUNSATURATED FATS** are considered to be one of the healthiest fats. They are found in nuts and high-fat fruits, such as olives and avocados.
- **SATURATED FATS,** such as coconut oil, butter and lard are stable and solidify when cold. They are found in full-cream (whole) milk products and in meat. Saturated fats are healthy when they come from natural sources and are used in moderation.
- **POLYUNSATURATED FATS** can be found mostly in seeds, seed oils and oily fish, such as salmon. For children, avoid larger fish that are higher up the food chain (see Fish and shellfish on page 38). Use non-hydrogenated, polyunsaturated fats from natural sources and in moderation. Margarine, although rich in polyunsaturated fats, is highly processed, often containing colours and additives.
- **OMEGA-3 FATTY ACIDS** are a type of polyunsaturated fat. These are very important for brain health and development. They're found in oily fish and seafood. Plant sources include chia seeds, linseeds (flax seeds), walnuts and macadamia nuts.
- **TRANS FATS** should be avoided, as they contribute to heart disease and inflammation in the body. Trans fats are often created when oils are partially hydrogenated to stabilise or harden them.

Fats recommended for you and your baby

Moderation is the key word with fats. Feed your family a creative mix of recipes so you enjoy the flavour variations that different fat levels create in foods, from steamed foods to stir-fries, and from light and fresh dishes to creamy sauces. Preferably use minimally processed fats and oils and avoid chemically treated hydrogenated oils that contain trans fats. Look for 'cold-pressed' or 'expeller-pressed' on the label, as these are the least processed. We recommend cooking using the following fats:

Nut oils

- Macadamia, hazelnut, almond or walnut
- Peanut

Seed oils

- Sunflower oil (high-oleic sunflower oil is healthiest and is higher in monunsaturates than other sunflower oils, but is harder to find at the supermarket), rice-bran oil or grapeseed oil

- Sesame oil (it's a delicious but strongly flavoured oil, so just a few drops is enough)

Other oils

- Olive oil
- Avocado oil
- Coconut oil (a natural saturated fat and a naturally sweet oil)

Dairy

- Butter
- Ghee, also known as clarified butter (it has the milk solids removed from it; it's rich in omega-3 and omega-9 fatty acids)

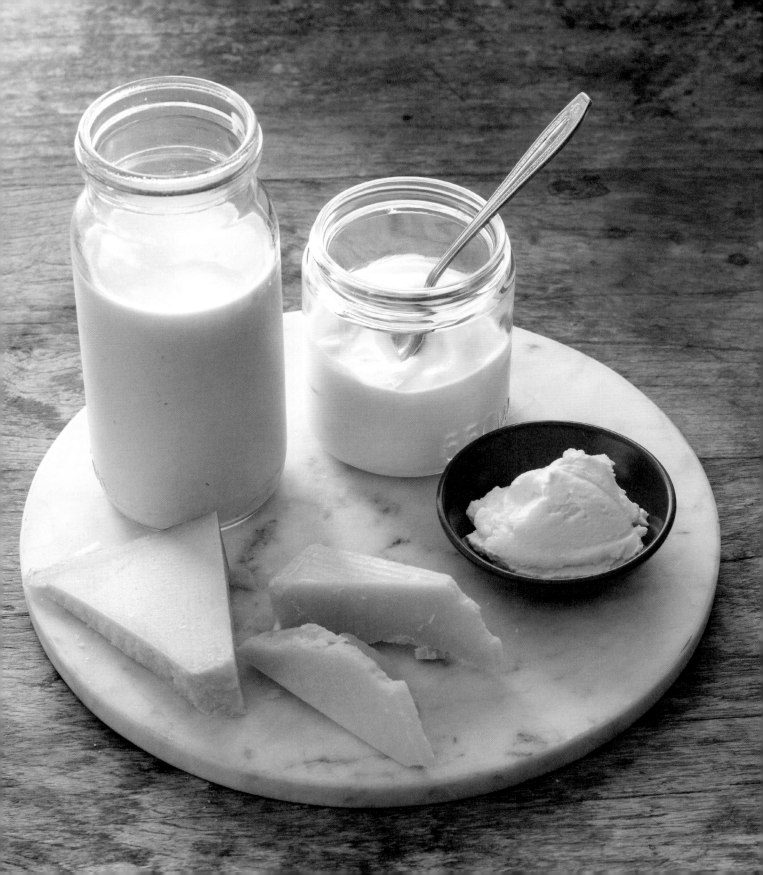

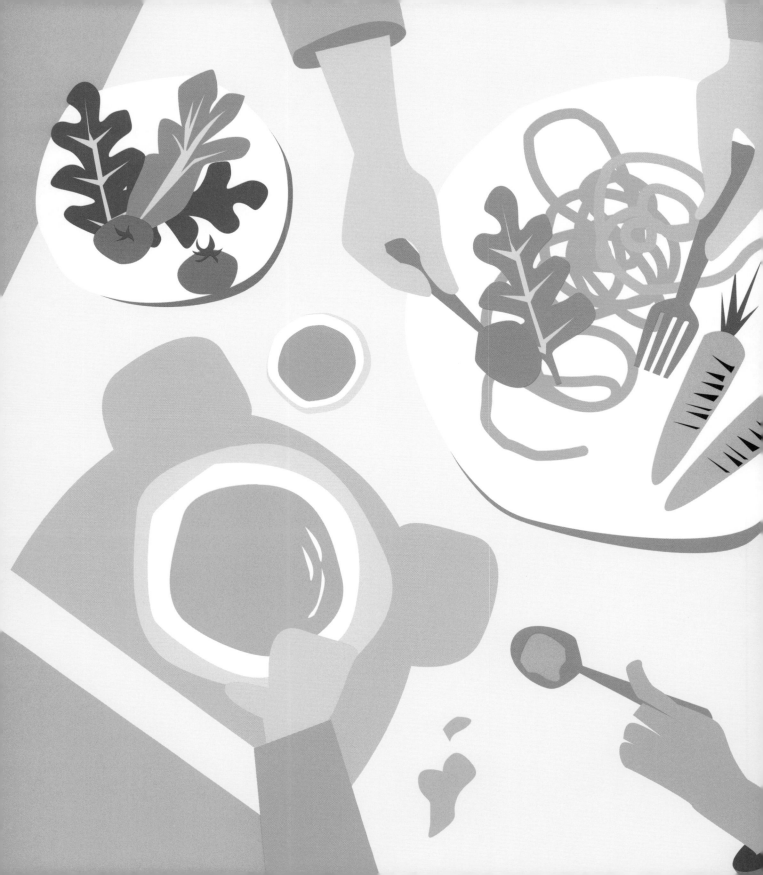

part two

The recipes

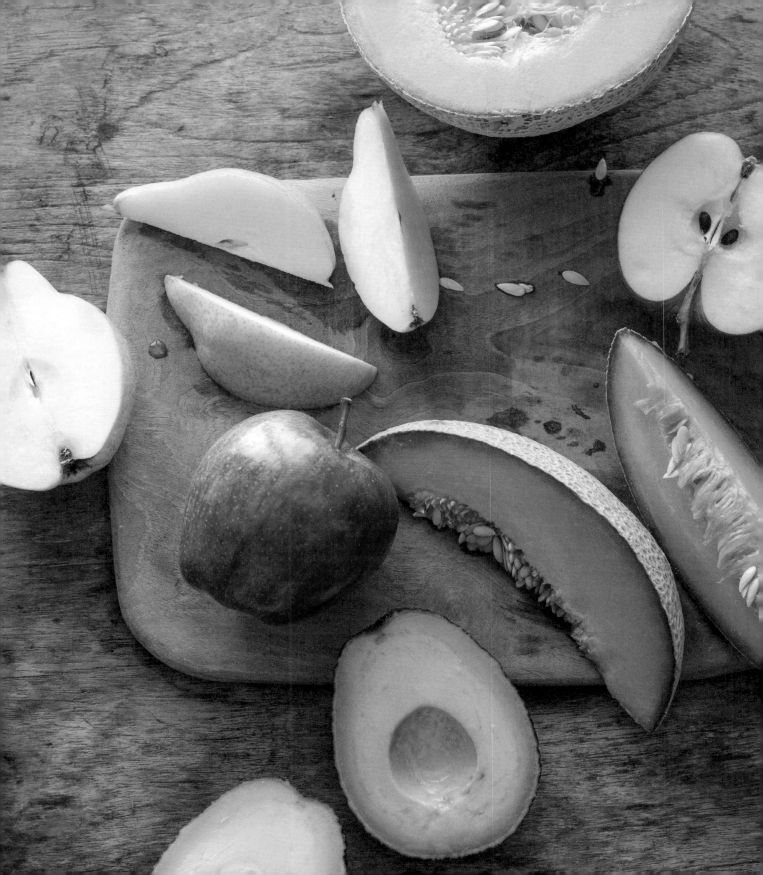

Important notes on the recipes

Plan your family's meals around fresh fruit and vegetables in season, and meats and fish that you can buy at the supermarket or farmers' markets. Also, keep the right dry ingredients and staples in your pantry to make easy, delicious and healthy recipes. You won't find nutritional balance within each recipe in this book, but you will find great meals that balance out over the week.

Allergens *are* included

So many children's foods today are labelled 'free from', which means they don't contain any food allergens. However, in this book we have taken the opposite approach and carefully and intentionally created recipes that do contain the common food allergens, showing you how to incorporate peanuts, tree nuts, eggs, dairy, wheat, fish, shellfish, soy and sesame into everyday family recipes. This makes it easy for you to include them in your baby's everyday diet. (To learn more about the common food allergens and how their early introduction may help prevent the development of food allergies in your child, see When and why to start introducing the common food allergens on page 34.)

Modifying the recipes for babies

Our recipes are created for the whole family to enjoy. However, most will require minor modifications to make them suitable for babies and toddlers, and this is clearly indicated in the recipes. The changes will usually relate to the texture of the dish, such as making a purée or mashing; not using salt for seasoning, or salty sauces; and reducing or omitting spicy ingredients.

Each recipe has a recommendation for preparation and serving for:

> **Younger babies** (6-9 months)
>
> **Older babies** (10-12 months)
>
> **Toddlers** (1-3 years)

No seasoning for baby's portion

You should not season your baby's food with salt for the first 12 months, as their kidneys cannot cope with excess salt. But these recipes are for the whole family so we have included seasoning instructions for older children and adults. We use salt cautiously in these recipes and recommend you set aside your baby's portion first, before seasoning to the adults' taste. Salty ingredients that you may want to omit altogether for babies under 12 months include:

- **Soy sauce**
- **Tamari**
- **Fish sauce**
- **Anchovies**
- **Miso**
- **Bacon and ham – if choosing bacon or ham always looked for naturally cured, nitrate-free**

Keep spices light

For younger babies, use a very light hand with spices to avoid tummy upsets, or omit them altogether. Some children are more tolerant to spices than others, so use your judgement. For older babies use a tiny amount of things such as pepper, cinnamon and other spices, and mustard. As your toddler's palate matures, very gradually increase the spice and eventually introduce the big flavours, such as chilli.

Sweet recipes

You'll see that most of the recipes are savoury. This is to encourage more adventurous eaters and introduce delicious flavours that aren't sweet - because babies tend to have a preference for sweet before 12 months. Save sweet meals such as desserts and snacks for occasional treats, and don't serve them every day. The slightly sweeter recipes in this section use maple syrup rather than honey. (Paediatricians recommend avoiding honey until after 12 months of age when your child's digestive system is more mature. Honey may contain spores of bacteria that can cause botulism.)

Serving sizes

The number of serves noted in the recipes is for older children and adults.

- **For baby, purée servings will start with a few teaspoons and build, depending on your baby's appetite and age, to ¼–1 cup as they approach 12 months.**

- **A toddler's serving size is usually about one-third to half of an adult's portion size.**

Avoid choking hazards

- **Watch your baby while they are eating to ensure they do not choke.**

- **Make sure your child is sitting still while eating.**

- **Make sure finger foods or mashed lumps in food for babies are in pea-sized pieces.**

- **Avoid foods that present a choking risk, such as nut chunks, whole grapes, chunky pieces of fruits, vegetables, sausage etc.**

- **Ensure that all bones are removed from fish or meat and that there aren't any sharp pieces in the food – such as the crusty bits from roast potatoes, or the sharp shards of poppadoms.**

- **Learn what to do if your child or an adult is choking so you can be prepared. There are useful first-aid references available on the internet, listed in the Notes section (see note 5).**

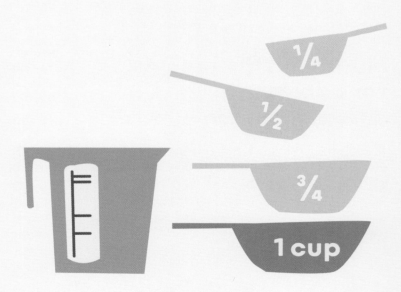

Substituting ingredients

When cooking at home, if you don't have an ingredient, you can swap it for what you do have. Most of our recipes include alternative options. Below are some suggested alternatives for common ingredients. However, note that if you change an ingredient in a recipe the allergens may also change.

INGREDIENT	ALTERNATIVE
Nut oils The common nut oils in the supermarket include peanut, almond, hazelnut, walnut and macadamia (this is our tree-nut oil of choice for baking, roasting, shallow frying and stir-frying. It has a delicious buttery flavour, contains more than 80% healthy monounsaturated fats, and has a high smoke point of 210°C (410°F)).	Another nut oil, or one of the following: olive oil, avocado oil, sunflower oil (high-oleic is the best), rice-bran oil or grapeseed oil *Ideally choose cold-pressed or expeller-pressed oils, as they are the least processed and a healthier choice.*
Milk Cow's or goat's	Coconut milk, soy milk, oat milk or nut milks, but always use unsweetened varieties
Cream	Full-fat coconut milk or coconut cream, or puréed silken tofu
Butter	Ghee
Fresh tomatoes	Tinned tomatoes
Fresh corn kernels	Frozen corn kernels
Dried beans and pulses	Tinned beans and pulses, but rinse and drain them

Allergen symbols

The recipes include symbols to denote which allergens are included in the ingredients (as well as any optional ingredients). Note that if you mix and match recipes, you will need to take note of the allergens within the recipe/ingredient you are adding.

Allergens

= **PEANUTS**

= **TREE NUTS**

= **EGGS**

= **DAIRY**

= **WHEAT**

= **SOY**

= **SESAME**

= **FISH**

= **SHELLFISH**

Kitchen tools

Having the right tools in your kitchen makes preparing family meals and baby food easy. If you're time poor, you'll want everything on hand so you can cook with the least effort and preferably in the shortest time possible. Below are our recommended utensils. Also note that oven temperatures in this book are for fan-forced ovens; if you are using a conventional oven, you may need to increase the temperature by 20°C (35°F) or adjust the cooking time.

Electric gadgets to make life easier

- **HAND-HELD, OR STICK, BLENDER** A hand-held electrical appliance for blending or puréeing small amounts of food in the pan or the container in which they are being prepared. These often come with various attachments, including a whisk, which is handy. Make sure you turn the blender off before removing it from the food or you'll redecorate your kitchen with the spray!

- **FOOD PROCESSOR** This electrical appliance for blending or puréeing food in bulk is ideal if you're preparing extra food to freeze.

- **ELECTRIC BEATERS** These are hand-held beaters that you can use to whisk, beat and whip. They are a cost-effective gadget to have on hand, especially if a larger food processor or free-standing mixer is out of your budget. The beaters are easy to clean – and fun for the kids to lick!

Optional

- **A BULLET BLENDER**, like the ones you use for making smoothies. It also works as a mini food processor.

- **A COFFEE/SPICE GRINDER** can also be very useful for small amounts of pesto, spice pastes or powders, but a solid mortar and pestle works well too and looks good in the kitchen.

Essential hand-held utensils

Hand-held utensils are a great way to get kids in the kitchen. Using these tools helps children understand the basics of cooking, such as stirring, folding, whisking, aerating and emulsifying.

- **LARGE SPOONS – SLOTTED OR PERFORATED** These are good for testing pasta, and safer for straining small amounts of steamed vegetables – instead of moving pots of boiling water from stovetop to sink (especially if there are toddlers at your feet).

- **LADLE** We find a 250 ml (8½ fl oz/1 cup) capacity ladle is most useful.

- **WOODEN SPOONS** Be sure to always wash these in very hot water to remove all food taints. Allow to dry thoroughly after use.

- **MEASURING SPOONS** This book uses 20 ml (¾ fl oz) tablespoons, so if you're working with 15 ml (½ fl oz) tablespoons be generous with your measurements.

- **MEASURING CUPS** Metric cup measurements are used in this book – 250 ml (8½ fl oz) for 1 cup. In the US, 1 cup is 237 ml (8 fl oz) so American cooks should be generous with their cup measurements. In the UK, 1 cup is 284 ml (9½ fl oz) so UK cooks should be scant with their measurements.

- **WHISK** A medium metal or plastic whisk is great – essential for omelettes and sauces.

- **RUBBER/SILICON SPATULA** Good for scraping ingredients out of bowls, but not for stirring hot pans or cooking at high temperatures, as the rubber can soften too much.

- **VEGETABLE PEELER** A garden-variety peeler, or alternatively a Y-peeler, is pretty vital to have on hand, and is much quicker than using a knife.

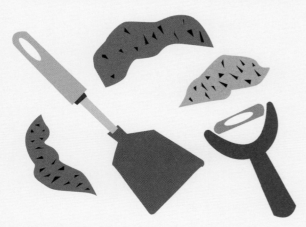

- **BOX GRATER** Used for shredding cheese or vegetables. The side of the box grater is useful for thin slicing if you do not have a mandoline (see below) and does all the things you need from a microplane too.

- **MANDOLINE** These are excellent for slicing ingredients very thinly – watch your fingers, though! You can get small hand-held versions or larger free-standing versions.

- **MICROPLANE** Ideal for grating parmesan cheese very finely. You can grate the cheese straight over the finished dish.

- **METAL MESH SIEVE** Essential for sifting and straining. Look for metal mesh and metal frame sieves, as they can take pressure without the mesh separating from the frame. It's handy to own two sieves – one small (12 cm/4¾ in diameter) for early baby food (and making loose-leaf tea!) and one medium (18 cm/7 in diameter).

Pans and other larger items

I'm still using my mother's baking trays, graters and enamelled pans. They're cooking heirlooms that I'm sure are more than 60 years old. If you buy quality items, they're sure to last a long time.

- **BAKING TINS** A couple of decent-sized, heavy, deep, metal roasting tins and a loaf (bar) tin will get you through.

- **BAKING/CASSEROLE DISHES** Ceramic dishes are great for pies and casseroles. If they're flameproof they can be transferred from stovetop to oven.

- **BAKING TRAYS/SHEETS** These are very shallow baking tins, useful for roasting nuts, cookies and other items. Lining baking trays with baking paper enables you to use less oil and reduces washing up. Shallow baking trays with a lip stop everything sliding off if you tip them.

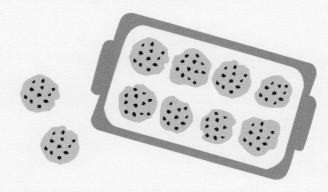

- **SAUCEPANS** Three heavy-based, stainless steel saucepans with lids – small, medium and large – will do for pretty much everything.

- **STEAMER** Get a good metal steamer with a lid that fits on top of your saucepans. Metal is best for baby food and is easy to keep clean.

- **MIXING BOWLS** Pyrex, glass, stainless steel or ceramic – a set of three sizes is ideal. Pyrex or glass is great for microwaving too.

- **LARGE COLANDER** You'll need this for draining pasta and larger-cut vegetables.

- **MEASURING JUG – PYREX OR PLASTIC** This is transparent, so it's easier to measure fluids and ensure it's clean.

- **CHOPPING BOARDS** Ideally use wood or plastic boards for cutting bread and vegetables (camphor wood boards are naturally antibacterial and great if you can get them) and plastic boards for raw meat and fish. Keep separate cutting boards for meat/fish and vegetables to prevent any cross-contamination from raw meats or seafood.

- **ICE-CUBE TRAYS** Trays of six large cubes are great for storing excess baby purées – you can get them in every shape, size and colour and with covers, too. (Of course you could even use them to make ice – pop an ice cube in a drink to help cope with family life!)

- **AIRTIGHT PLASTIC CONTAINERS** These are great for storing leftovers and snacks. Buy freezer-safe containers for freezing food. Sealable zip-lock bags are also ideal for storing food for freezing. You can freeze food in portioned sizes.

- **FRYING PANS** We recommend cast-iron, seasoned frying pans.

TEFLON-COATED NON-STICK PANS

Until 2015, Teflon pans contained perfluorooctanoic acid (PFOA), which was a health concern. These days non-stick pans are PFOA-free, but there are a few important tips for safe use:

- **Teflon pans should only be used on low to medium heat.**

- **Damaged or scratched Teflon-coated pans should be discarded.**

- **To avoid overheating, don't heat an empty pan.**

- **Use only wooden or silicon utensils on non-stick pans to avoid scratching.**

- **Hand-wash teflon pans with a soft cloth rather than scouring pads or steel wool, which can scratch.**

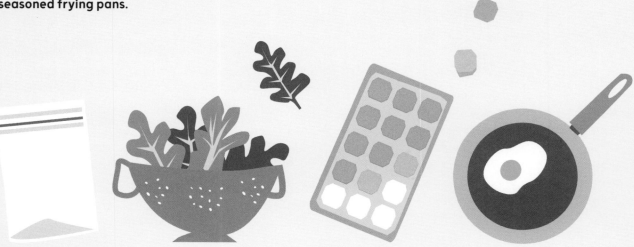

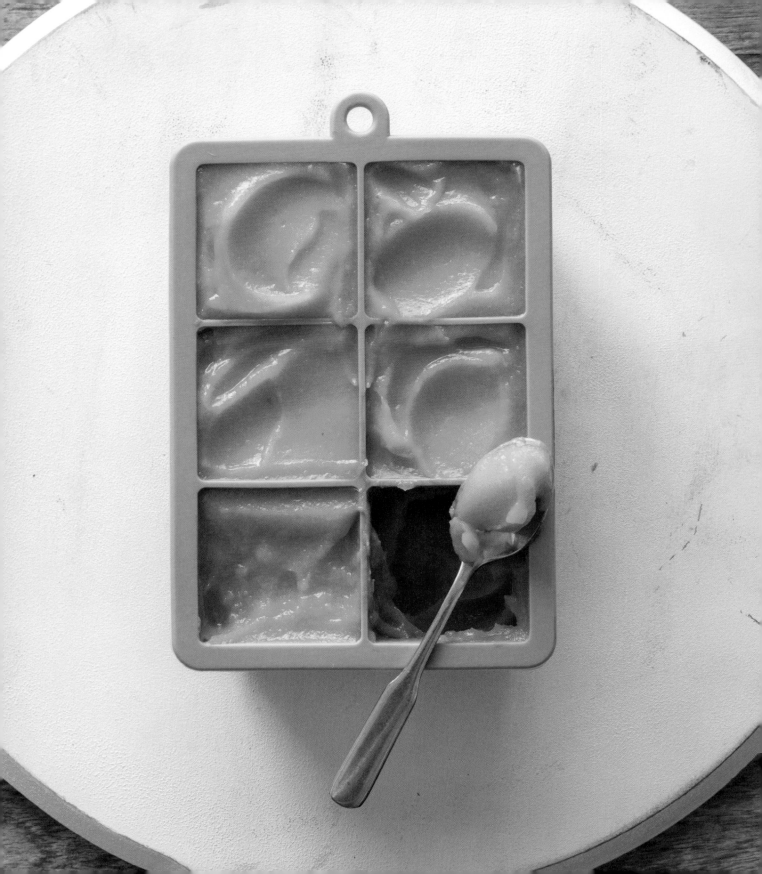

breakfast

BABY'S FIRST CEREAL

OPTIONAL

It's so easy to make a flavourful, healthy first cereal for baby at home. All you need is a quality, high-speed food processor or blender. This cereal combines three nutritious grains and is easy for your baby to digest. Brown rice crumbs are available in health or organic food stores – or you can grind up rice cakes, but only use those that list the ingredients as 100 per cent rice.

Nuts are optional in this recipe. You can add nuts to the dry ingredients when processing the cereal in the blender, or make up your cereal without nuts and serve the prepared cereal with ¼ teaspoon of a smooth, unsalted nut butter (see Home-made nut butters on page 217).

60 g (2 oz/1 cup) brown rice crumbs
50 g (1¾ oz/¾ cup) organic amaranth
flakes (or quinoa flakes)
35 g (1¼ oz/¼ cup) oat bran
1 teaspoon almonds, or nuts of choice,
coarsely chopped (optional)
1½ tablespoons warm boiled water,
warm breast milk or formula, to serve
fruit or vegetable purée, such as
carrot, banana or red apple, to serve
(optional)
smooth, unsalted nut butter, to serve
(optional)

Add the brown rice crumbs, amaranth flakes, oat bran and the coarsely chopped nuts, if using, to a blender and process until fine and smooth with no lumps or coarse pieces. Pass your ground dry cereal through a sieve to ensure the mixture is as smooth as possible.

Put the warm boiled water, breast milk or formula into a small bowl and sprinkle over 1 tablespoon of the cereal. Whisk with a fork for 30 seconds to prevent any lumps from forming, then allow to rest for 2-3 minutes, stirring occasionally. The cereal should be smooth and creamy.

Serve with a little fruit or vegetable purée and add ¼ teaspoon nut butter for a richer flavour, if desired. Always check the temperature before serving.

Store any unused dry cereal in an airtight container in the refrigerator for up to 30 days.

NOTE: Gradually increase the serving size as your baby (and their appetite) grows.

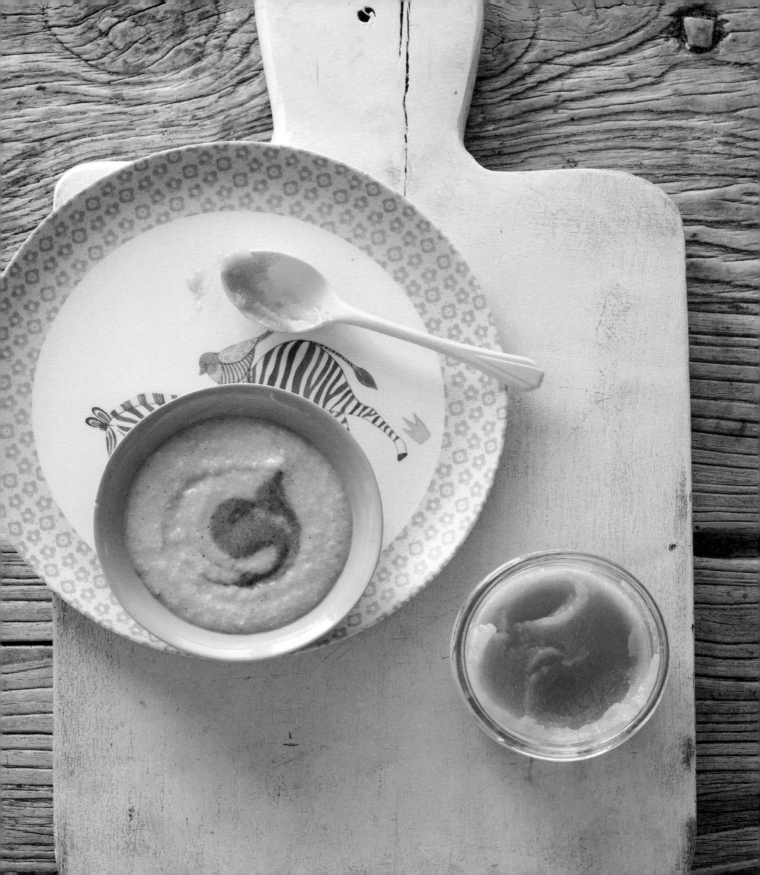

CLASSIC BIRCHER

SERVES 4–6

PREP TIME: 5 MINUTES,
PLUS OVERNIGHT SOAKING

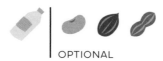

OPTIONAL

Soaking oats in yoghurt and fruit juice overnight softens and breaks down the grains, making a delicious, fibre-rich, easily digestible probiotic breakfast for the whole family. To add nuts, consider folding a little smooth, unsalted nut butter (see Home-made nut butters on page 217) through your bircher or, for a dairy-free alternative, swap out regular yoghurt for a coconut, soy or nut-milk yoghurt. You will need to start your bircher a day ahead so the oats are well soaked.

100 g (3¼ oz/1 cup) rolled (porridge) oats

250 ml (8½ fl oz/1 cup) cloudy apple juice

250 g (9 oz/1 cup) Greek-style or full-fat plain yoghurt

Powernut crumble (page 221), to serve (optional)

fresh fruit, to serve (optional)

Mix the oats together with the apple juice and yoghurt. Cover and soak overnight in the refrigerator. To serve, add a good sprinkling of powernut crumble and fresh fruit, if desired.

Store in a sealed container in the refrigerator for up to 3 days.

> **For younger babies** purée the bircher and crumble until smooth and silky - if the purée is too thick add a little extra water or milk.
>
> **For older babies** serve the bircher as is, but blitz the crumble to a fine crumb. Serve with coarsely mashed fruit, if desired.
>
> **For toddlers** serve as for adults with fresh berries, if desired. If using the Powernut crumble, make sure the nuts and seeds are finely chopped.

Variations

There are endless great ideas for variations on classic bircher, as well as garnishes, such as nuts (pecans are a favourite), seeds, fresh and poached fruits, spices and assorted grains.

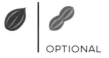

OPTIONAL

ALMOND MILK BERRY BIRCHER

To make a berry bircher using almond milk instead of regular yoghurt, mix the oats in a bowl with ½ cup mixed fresh or frozen berries. Add 500 ml (17 fl oz/2 cups) almond milk to coat the oats well (add a little extra if required) and mix well. Cover and soak overnight in the refrigerator. The next day, add the juice of 1 lemon and a pinch of ground cinnamon (just a tiny amount for babies) to the oats and mix well. This is great served with coconut yoghurt, extra fresh berries and chopped nuts.

For younger babies purée the bircher and toppings until smooth.

For older babies lightly mash the bircher with a fork to soften any lumps or clumps. If adding coconut and chopped nuts, blitz them into fine pieces in a blender or food processor.

For toddlers serve as for adults with fresh berries. If adding chopped nuts, grind them into coarse/small pieces in a blender or food processor, or chop finely.

OPTIONAL

ALMOND MILK QUINOA BIRCHER

Combine 155 g (5½ oz/2 cups) quinoa flakes in a bowl with 65 g (2¼ oz/½ cup) LSA meal, 30 g (1 oz/½ cup) shredded coconut, 70 g (2½ oz/½ cup) pepitas (pumpkin seeds), 80 g (2¾ oz/½ cup) chopped almonds, a pinch of ground cinnamon (just a tiny amount for babies), 1 teaspoon natural vanilla extract, 250 ml (8½ fl oz/1 cup) fresh orange juice and 500 ml (17 fl oz/2 cups) almond milk. Mix well, cover and soak overnight in the refrigerator. The next day, mix again and serve with flaked coconut, chopped almonds and a little orange zest.

For younger babies purée the bircher and toppings until smooth.

For older babies purée the bircher and toppings to a coarse texture, then sprinkle with orange zest. If topping with nuts or seeds, grind them into a fine crumb in a blender or food processor.

For toddlers serve as for adults, but if adding chopped nuts grind them into fine pieces in a blender or food processor.

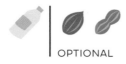

OPTIONAL

RICE AND MILLET BIRCHER

Take 75 g (2¾ oz/1 cup) rice flakes and 75 g (2¾ oz/1 cup) millet flakes (if no millet flakes are available, use 75 g/2¾ oz/½ cup instant polenta) and soak them in 250 ml (8½ fl oz/1 cup) apple juice mixed with 250 ml (8½ fl oz/1 cup) water. Cover and soak overnight in the refrigerator. The next day add 500 g (1 lb 2 oz/ 2 cups) plain unsweetened yoghurt and your favourite toppings - a dusting of LSA meal or berries, nuts and shredded coconut are all great options.

For younger babies purée the bircher and toppings until smooth.

For older babies purée the bircher and toppings to a coarse texture. If topping with nuts or seeds, grind them into a fine crumb in a blender or food processor.

For toddlers serve as for adults, but if adding nuts grind them into fine pieces in a blender or food processor.

NOTE: LSA meal is a mixture of ground linseeds (flax seeds), sunflower seeds and almonds.

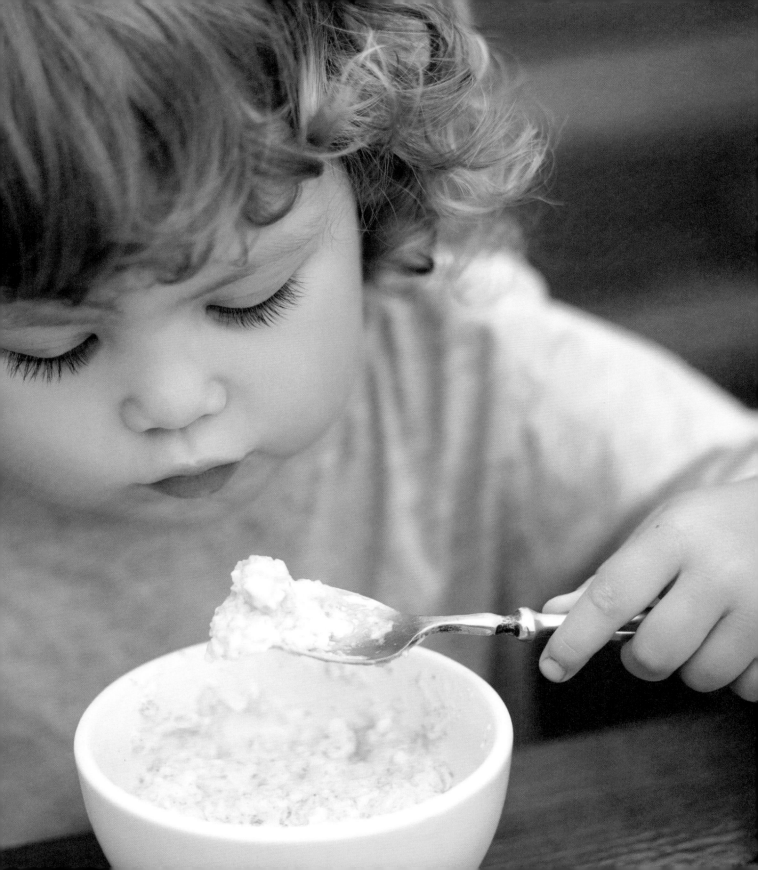

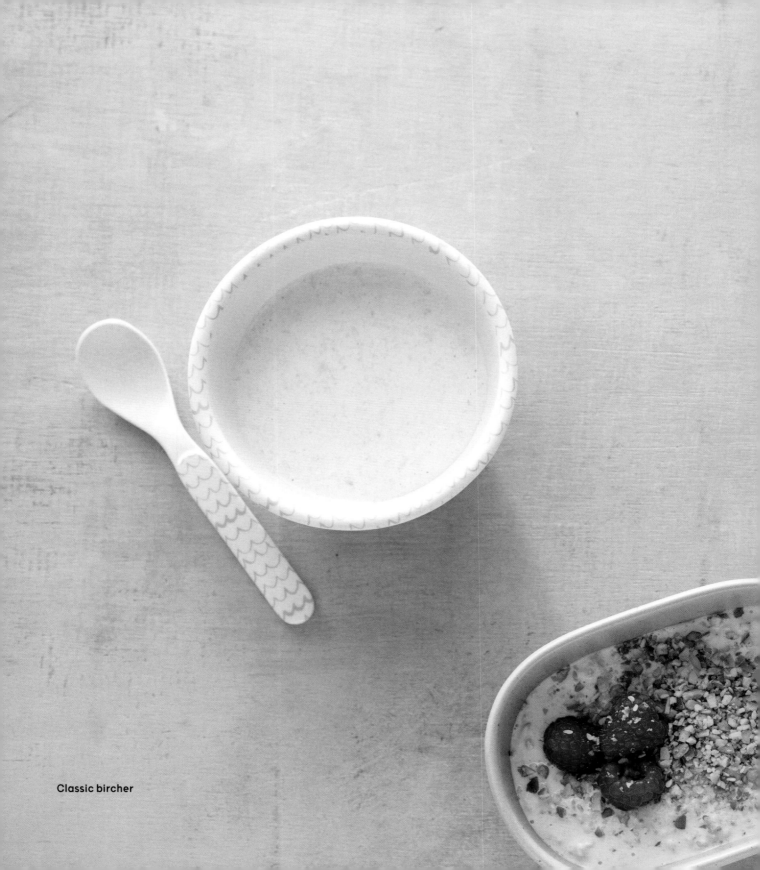

Classic bircher

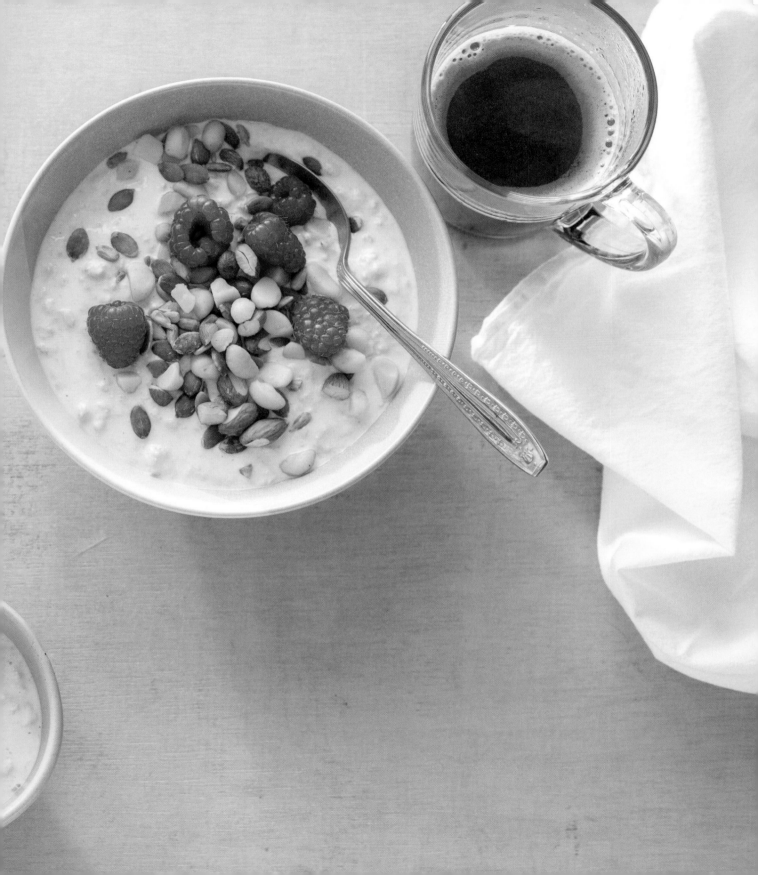

CLASSIC PORRIDGE

SERVES 4

PREP TIME: 2 MINUTES

COOKING TIME: 8 MINUTES

OPTIONAL

This recipe is an ideal base for adding optional nuts and seeds – especially if making your porridge with water. Feel free to swap the cow's milk for almond, macadamia or soy milk and add fruit – poached, roasted or stewed – with just a touch of cinnamon (just a tiny amount for babies). We love serving porridge with apples roasted in maple syrup, and topped with pecans. Warm cooked oats provide a slow release of energy to sustain you until lunchtime. Legendary chef Nigel Slater (who only cooks his porridge with water) suggests letting your porridge set into cakes and then frying them in butter.

160 g (5½ oz) rolled (porridge) oats
600 ml (20½ fl oz) milk or water
tiny pinch of salt

Place the oats and milk or water in a medium saucepan over medium heat. Add the salt, then as soon as you see your first 'bubble' stir with a wooden spoon. (Traditionalists will tell you to only stir clockwise!) Bring to a gentle simmer and continue to cook and stir for about 5 minutes until you have a beautiful creamy porridge. You can adjust the consistency to your liking by simply adding a little more milk or water for a sightly runnier porridge. Serve immediately, as the porridge thickens quickly once rested. Store in a sealed container in the refrigerator for up to 3 days.

> **For younger babies** purée the porridge until smooth and allow to cool before serving. Serve topped with puréed fruits, if desired. To add nuts, stir in ¾ teaspoon of a smooth, unsalted nut butter of your choice (see Home-made nut butters on page 217).
>
> **For older babies** serve as is or topped with mashed stewed fruits, and allow to cool before serving. If adding nuts, grind them into fine pieces in a blender or food processor.
>
> **For toddlers** serve as for adults, but make sure any added nuts and seeds are finely chopped. Allow to cool before serving.

OPTIONAL

QUINOA AND ALMOND PORRIDGE

Place 100 g (3½ oz / ½ cup) well rinsed quinoa in a saucepan and cover with 250 ml (8½ fl oz / 1 cup) water. Bring to the boil, then simmer until most of the water has been absorbed. Add 250 ml (8½ fl oz / 1 cup) almond milk, a pinch of ground cinnamon (only a tiny amount for babies) and 1 teaspoon natural vanilla extract. Heat, stirring, until the quinoa is creamy. Stir through 35 g (1¼ oz / ¼ cup) Powernut crumble (page 221) to serve, if desired. Store in a sealed container in the refrigerator for up to 3 days.

> **For younger babies** purée the porridge and toppings until smooth and allow to cool before serving.
>
> **For older babies** serve as is and allow to cool before serving. If adding the powernut crumble, process it into coarse crumbs in a blender or food processor.
>
> **For toddlers** serve as for adults, but make sure the powernut crumble is finely chopped. Allow to cool before serving.

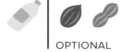

OPTIONAL

BUCKWHEAT PORRIDGE

To make buckwheat porridge, swap the oats for buckwheat (you will need to cover the buckwheat with water and let it soak overnight - rinse and drain in the morning), then follow the method for classic porridge. Store in a sealed container in the refrigerator for up to 3 days.

> **For younger babies** purée the porridge until smooth and allow to cool before serving. Top with fruit purée or stir through ¼ teaspoon of a smooth, unsalted nut butter (see Home-made nut butters on page 217).
>
> **For older babies** serve as is and allow to cool before serving. Top with mashed stewed fruits. If adding nuts, process them into fine pieces in a blender or food processor.
>
> **For toddlers** serve as for adults, or topped with mashed stewed fruits. If adding nuts, grind them into fine pieces in a blender or food processor. Allow to cool before serving.

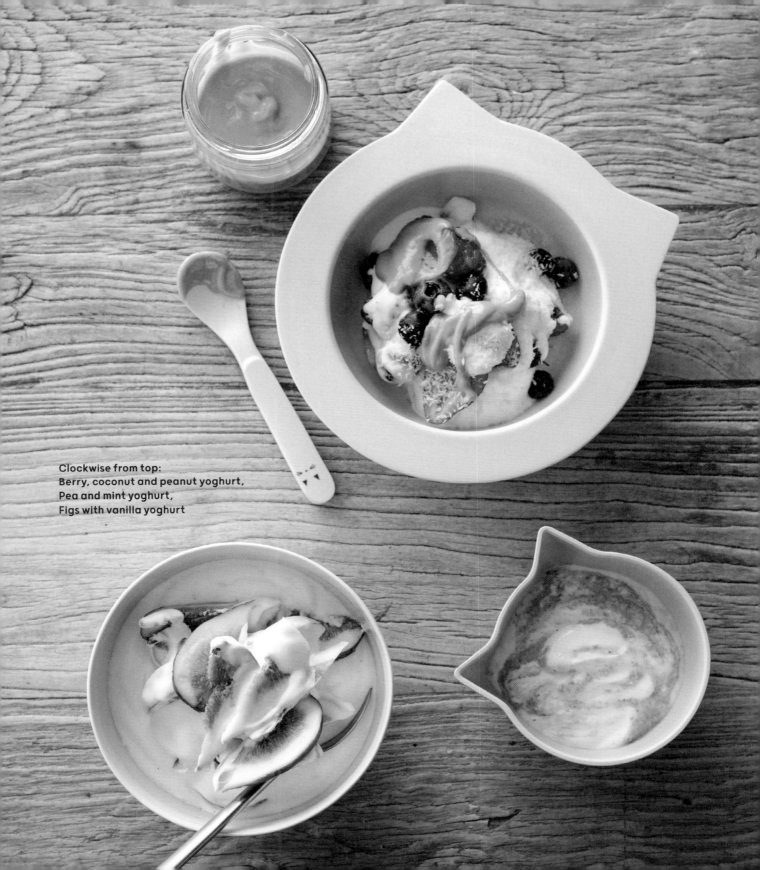

Clockwise from top:
Berry, coconut and peanut yoghurt,
Pea and mint yoghurt,
Figs with vanilla yoghurt

YOGHURTS

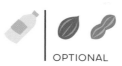

OPTIONAL

Yoghurt is a naturally fermented, calcium-rich food and makes a delicious start to the day. The flavour options are countless. For dairy yoghurt always buy full-fat yoghurt made only from milk and cultures, with no added sugar or artificial additives. We often use Greek-style yoghurt, which is strained to make it even thicker and creamier.

500 g (1 lb 2 oz/2 cups) Greek-style or
   full-fat plain yoghurt
½ teaspoon natural vanilla extract

SIMPLE VANILLA YOGHURT

Simply mix the yoghurt and vanilla together, and this will give you a tasty base for the breakfast yoghurt variations that follow. The added vanilla also makes this a lovely dessert. Store in a sealed container in the refrigerator for up to 3 days.

> **For younger babies** yoghurts are a more concentrated source of the dairy proteins, so for baby's first foods make sure you serve the yoghurt with fruit or vegetable purées for balance.
>
> **For older babies** serve topped with mashed fruits and finely ground nuts or seeds.
>
> **For toddlers** serve as for adults, topped with fruits and finely chopped nuts or seeds, if desired.

Variations

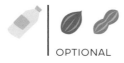

OPTIONAL

FIGS WITH VANILLA YOGHURT

Gently cut 4 figs into thin slices or small wedges and fold them through the vanilla yoghurt. Add a drop or two of hazelnut oil to jazz it up, if desired. Store in a sealed container in the refrigerator for up to 3 days.

> **For younger babies** purée the yoghurt and figs until silky smooth.
>
> **For older babies** purée the yoghurt and figs to a slightly lumpy consistency, or slice the figs thinly for a first finger food.
>
> **For toddlers** serve as for adults.

BERRY, COCONUT AND PEANUT YOGHURT

Mix together 500 g (1 lb 2 oz/2 cups) vanilla yoghurt, 1 cup of seasonal berries (blueberries, strawberries, blackberries and raspberries are all wonderful here), 25 g (1 oz/¼ cup) toasted desiccated coconut and 2 tablespoons smooth, unsalted peanut butter (see Home-made nut butters on page 217). Store in a sealed container in the refrigerator for up to 3 days.

> **For younger babies** purée all the ingredients until silky smooth.
>
> **For older babies** mash the fruits to a soft lumpy texture and serve with vanilla yoghurt and smooth, unsalted peanut butter.
>
> **For toddlers** serve as for adults.

OPTIONAL

POWERFOOD PINK BREAKFAST BOWL

Take 500 g (1 lb 2 oz/2 cups) vanilla yoghurt and add it to a food processor with 2 cups of seasonal red fruit (any berries - dragon fruit is also perfect here). Purée lightly to blend in the fruits. Just for the adults, add an optional 2 tablespoons protein powder. Serve sprinkled with a little Powernut crumble (page 221) and extra fresh berries. Store in a sealed container in the refrigerator for up to 2 days.

> **For younger babies** purée all the ingredients until silky smooth.
>
> **For older babies** blitz the powernut crumble into a fine crumb and sprinkle over the yoghurt to serve.
>
> **For toddlers** blitz the powernut crumble into coarse pieces and sprinkle over the yoghurt with some fresh berries.

DATE AND WALNUT YOGHURT

Mix together 500 g (1 lb 2 oz / 2 cups) vanilla yoghurt, 50 g (1¾ oz / ½ cup) toasted walnuts and 90 g (3 oz / ½ cup) pitted dates. Cover and soak overnight in the refrigerator to soften the nuts and dates. Serve with a sprinkling of ground cinnamon (just a tiny amount for babies). For the adults, drizzle with maple syrup or dark agave syrup to serve. Store in a sealed container in the refrigerator for up to 3 days.

> **For younger babies** purée everything until smooth.
>
> **For older babies** process to a soft lumpy texture.
>
> **For toddlers** blitz briefly to break down the walnuts to finely chopped pieces.

Plain yoghurt variations

LEMON MYRTLE MACADAMIA YOGHURT

Lemon myrtle is a delicious Australian bushfood. If you can find it, mix ½ teaspoon dried lemon myrtle through 500 g (1 lb 2 oz / 2 cups) plain yoghurt. If you can't access lemon myrtle, substitute 1 teaspoon grated lemon zest. Leave to infuse overnight. Add 150 g (5½ oz / ½ cup) smooth, unsalted macadamia butter (see Home-made nut butters on page 217) or finely chopped raw or toasted macadamia nuts and mix well. To serve, top with a small drizzle of maple syrup to balance the tartness of the lemon. Store in a sealed container in the refrigerator for up to 2 days.

> **For younger babies** purée everything until smooth.
>
> **For older babies** serve as is, but if using macadamia nuts grind them into fine pieces in a blender or food processor.
>
> **For toddlers** serve as for adults, but ensure that the macadamia nuts are finely chopped.

>

PEA AND MINT YOGHURT

This is a great lunch idea for small people. It also makes a savoury yoghurt for all the family, or you can serve it as a delicious sauce with lamb chops, chicken skewers or roast vegies. Purée the following ingredients using a hand-held blender: 155 g (5½ oz/1 cup) defrosted frozen peas, 1 tablespoon olive oil, 1 teaspoon roughly chopped fresh mint, a pinch of salt (omit for babies) and a little freshly ground black pepper (just a tiny amount for babies). Fold through 250 g (9 oz/1 cup) Greek-style yoghurt. Blend to the desired consistency for adults. Store in a sealed container in the refrigerator for up to 2 days.

> **For younger babies** purée everything until smooth and serve a dollop on top of some plain yoghurt.
>
> **For older babies** serve as is or with mashed roast vegies.
>
> **For toddlers** serve as for adults.

REAL BAKED BEANS

SERVES 6

PREP TIME: 10 MINUTES

COOKING TIME: 55 MINUTES

OPTIONAL

This is a wonderful recipe for all ages, and a source of delicious plant proteins. Feel free to swap the white beans for any tinned beans you like – borlotti (cranberry) beans are great. The beans are delicious served with a soft fried egg on top (for older children and adults).

1 tablespoon macadamia oil

150 g (5¼ oz) naturally smoked bacon, coarsely chopped (omit for babies)

1 brown onion, finely diced

2 garlic cloves, finely chopped (just a tiny amount for babies)

3 large tomatoes, roughly chopped

2 tablespoons tomato paste (concentrated purée)

125 ml (4 fl oz/½ cup) maple syrup

1 teaspoon dijon mustard or ¼ teaspoon mustard powder (just a tiny amount for babies)

3 tablespoons red-wine vinegar or sherry vinegar

375 ml (12¼ fl oz/1½ cups) quality vegetable stock (preferably preservative and additive free) or water

800 g (1 lb 12 oz) tinned white beans (cannellini or haricot are fine), rinsed and drained

butter, to serve

sea salt (omit for babies)

freshly ground black pepper (just a tiny amount for babies)

Heat the macadamia oil in a large saucepan over medium heat. Add the bacon and fry, stirring, for about 2 minutes. Add the onion and garlic and continue cooking until they are soft. Add the tomatoes, tomato paste, maple syrup, mustard, vinegar and stock and bring gently to the boil. Add the beans, reduce the heat to very low and leave to simmer, uncovered, for about 45 minutes, until the sauce is thick and the beans are well coated – add a little water during cooking if the mixture is too thick.

Before serving, fold through a small amount of butter to add gloss and richness. Season with salt and pepper to taste. Store in a sealed container in the refrigerator for up to 3 days.

For younger babies purée until smooth and allow to cool before serving. If topping with an egg, purée a well-cooked hard-boiled egg.

For older babies purée to a lumpy texture and allow to cool before serving. Top with half a finely chopped hard-boiled egg, if desired.

For toddlers serve as for adults, but allow to cool before serving.

BUBBLE AND SQUEAK

SERVES 6-8

PREP TIME: 5 MINUTES

COOKING TIME: 8 MINUTES

OPTIONAL

Kitchen recycling? Bottom of the refrigerator breakfast or dinner? Whatever you choose to call it, bubble and squeak is not only delicious but makes great sense. Use leftovers and some of those vegetables that are still fresh but don't quite make the salad grade. Roasted or steamed left-over vegies are easy to digest, and add extra flavour. We love our bubble and squeak served with soft scrambled eggs (make sure they're thoroughly cooked through for children under 2) and often cook a little diced ham (omit for babies) through it as well.

8 medium cooked potatoes, mashed
    roughly with a fork (or use any
    left-over cooked root vegetable,
    e.g. carrot, pumpkin/squash,
    swede/ rutabaga)
an equal volume of shredded greens,
    such as kale, English spinach,
    cabbage or chard
sea salt (omit for babies)
freshly ground black pepper (just a tiny
    amount for babies)
1 tablespoon plain (all-purpose) flour
    (substitute with gluten-free flour
    if family members are gluten-
    intolerant or coeliac)
40 g (1½ oz) ghee, butter or nut oil

Mix the potatoes and greens together in a large bowl and season lightly with salt and pepper. Mix through the flour.

Place a medium-large frying pan over medium-high heat and add a good dollop of ghee, butter or your nut oil of choice. When the pan is hot add the vegetables. Press the mixture down firmly with a spoon, reduce the heat slightly and cook for a further 2 minutes without touching - you want a nice crust to form underneath. Carefully fold the bubble and squeak over in large sections so the crusty bottom comes to the top. Cook for a further 2 minutes, then serve.

Store in a sealed container in the refrigerator for up to 24 hours.

> **For younger babies** thin the mixture with a tablespoon of water or milk of your choice before puréeing until smooth. Allow to cool before serving.
>
> **For older babies** add a tablespoon of water or milk of your choice and mash to a lumpy texture. Allow to cool before serving.
>
> **For toddlers** chop into pieces and allow to cool before serving.

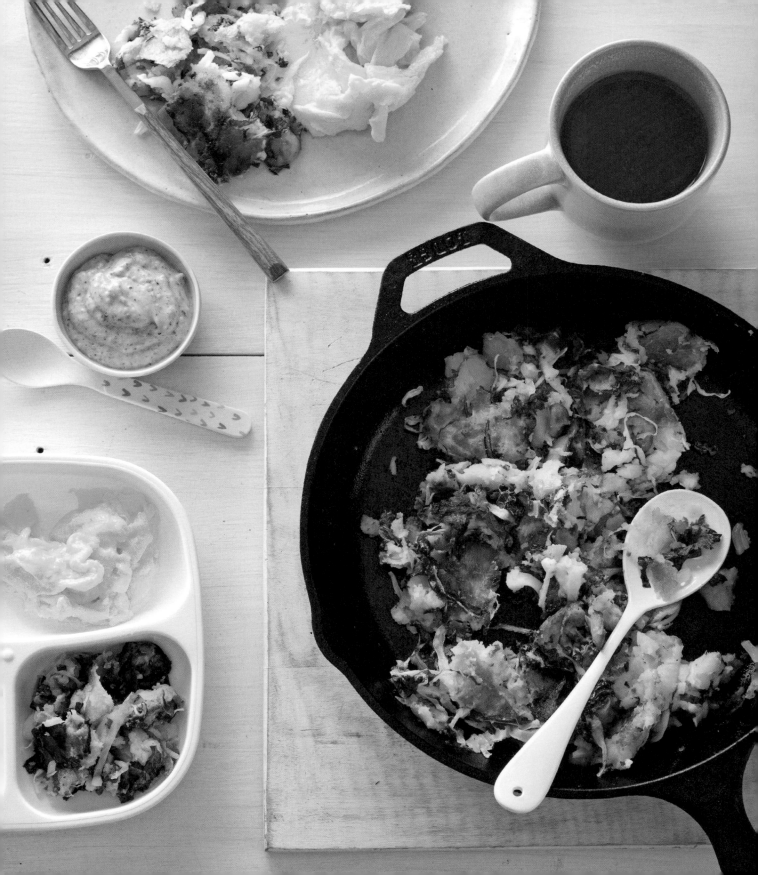

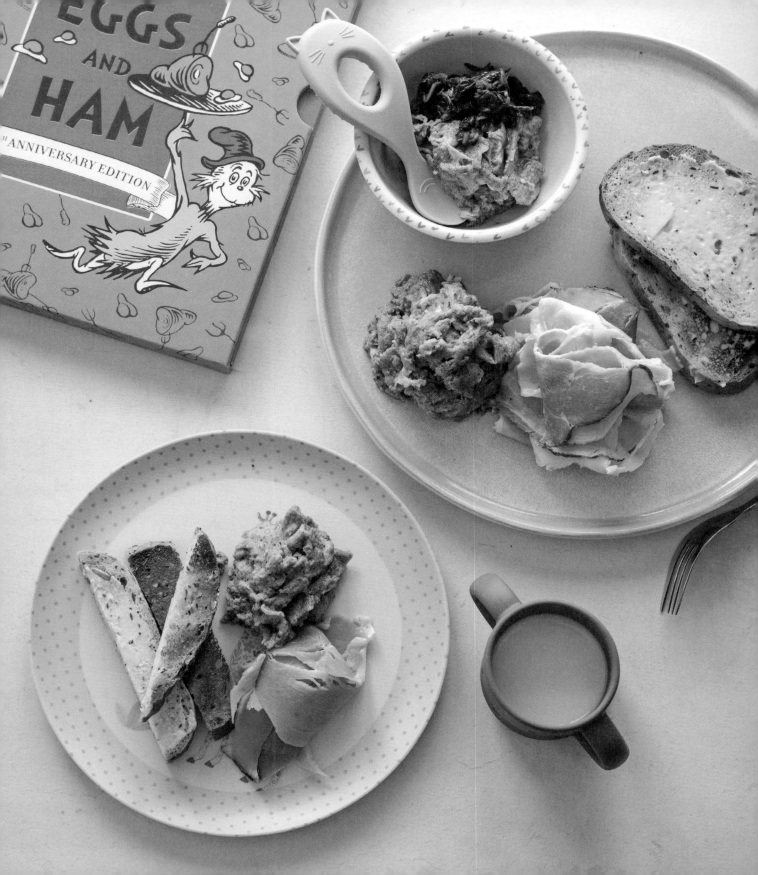

GREEN EGGS AND HAM

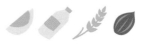

Straight out of the pages of the famous Dr Seuss book, this is a truly delicious savoury breakfast for kids of all ages. It also introduces toddlers and children to colourful dishes with new flavours. Pesto can be a strong flavour for young babies, so it's best to substitute wilted spinach in this dish.

6 eggs
2 tablespoons pouring (single/light) cream or yoghurt
40 g (1½ oz) Basil pesto (page 202)
40 g (1 ½ oz) butter, plus extra for the toast
4 slices quality bread (preferably sourdough), toasted
8 slices quality ham (omit for babies)

WILTED SPINACH
1 teaspoon butter or olive oil
large handful of English spinach

If making wilted spinach to use instead of pesto, heat the butter or oil in a small saucepan over medium heat. Add the spinach, cover the pan with a lid, reduce the heat to low and leave the spinach to wilt for 2 minutes. Set aside.

Lightly beat the eggs and cream or yoghurt together using a fork, then stir through the pesto or wilted spinach.

Melt the butter in a heavy frying pan over medium heat. Just as the butter starts to bubble, add the egg mixture and cook, folding gently (not robustly stirring), for about 2 minutes, or until you have perfectly soft, folded eggs. (For babies cook the eggs until firm.) Serve the eggs on buttered toast and curl the ham beside it, if desired.

> **For younger babies** add a tablespoon or two of yoghurt or milk to the well-cooked egg and spinach mixture, then purée until smooth. Allow to cool before serving.
>
> **For older babies** mash the well-cooked egg mixture to a slightly lumpy texture (add a little yoghurt or milk if it's too lumpy) and allow to cool before serving. Serve with finely chopped wilted spinach on the side.
>
> **For toddlers** cut the bread into 'soldiers' (finger-sized pieces), and chop the egg up. Allow to cool before serving.

OMELETTES

SERVES 1-2

PREP TIME: 5 MINUTES

COOKING TIME: 5 MINUTES

There is nothing more simple or delicious than an omelette, and it makes a super-quick breakfast (or lunch or dinner for that matter). You can vary the fillings – try chopped tomato and avocado with fresh coriander (cilantro); ricotta and spinach; sautéed mushrooms, gruyére cheese and chopped fresh parsley; or Bubble and squeak (page 74). Make sure your filling is cooked and ready to go before you start making the actual omelette. If you are cooking for the whole family, make a large omelette with double the ingredients below and cut it into portions – if you need more, a second one is only minutes away! If you are using ricotta for babies, you may like to use the recipe for Home-made ricotta on page 218.

20 g (¾ oz) butter
2–3 eggs, beaten together with
    1 tablespoon water (this makes the
    omelette fluffier)
sea salt (omit for babies)
freshly ground black pepper (just a tiny
    amount for babies)
1 tablespoon grated parmesan (use
    ricotta for babies)

BASIC OMELETTE

Place a heavy-based frying pan - or a special omelette pan if you have one - over medium-high heat. Add the butter and allow it to bubble and start to turn nutty brown.

Add the cooked (or raw) filling of your choice. Toss for a minute to warm the filling through, then add the egg mixture.

Keep the omelette moving in the pan by stirring the eggs from the outside of the pan to the centre using a rubber spatula. (Set aside baby's portion now and return it to the pan later to ensure that the eggs are fully cooked through.)

When the egg is still a little soft, add some salt and pepper and sprinkle the parmesan across the entire surface of the omelette. Fold one-third of the omelette into the centre using the spatula, then the other third over to cover the ingredients. Turn the omelette out onto a board by inverting the pan.

If you want to leave the omelette whole and round, another idea is to finish it under a grill (broiler) so it becomes a bit more frittata-esque. Serve hot. Store in a sealed container in the refrigerator for up to 2 days.

> **For younger babies** add a little milk to some chopped omelette and purée until smooth.
>
> **For older babies and toddlers** cut the omelette into thin strips for ideal finger food. Ensure any added fillings are finely chopped.

Variation

SERVES 1

GREEN OMELETTE

In a blender or food processor, combine 2 or 3 eggs and a pinch of salt (omit for babies) with a small handful of baby English spinach and blend until smooth and fluffy. Add the green egg mixture to the pan at the bubbling butter stage and cook as per the method opposite. When the egg is still a touch undercooked, add a further 15 g (½ oz / ¼ cup) spinach leaves along with a tiny pinch of ground turmeric. Season. Sprinkle parmesan (or ricotta for babies) over the surface of the omelette, then serve as per the method opposite.

> **For younger babies** add a little milk to some chopped omelette and purée until smooth.
>
> **For older babies and toddlers** cut the omelette into thin strips for ideal finger food.

SWEET CORN AND MACADAMIA FRITTERS

SERVES 4

PREP TIME: 10 MINUTES

COOKING TIME: 5 MINUTES

OPTIONAL

Flavourful and fast and easy to prepare, these fritters are a favourite to share with family and friends over breakfast or brunch. If you have time to make it, serve with Tuscan-style salad with buffalo mozzarella (page 99) to transform this into a truly special meal.

160 g (5¼ oz/1 cup) roasted macadamia nuts
kernels from 3 large corn cobs
1 small red onion, roughly chopped
2 eggs
¼ bunch coriander (cilantro), leaves and stems roughly chopped
sea salt (omit for babies)
freshly ground black pepper (just a tiny amount for babies)
150 g (5¼ oz/1 cup) plain (all-purpose) flour (substitute gluten-free flour if family members are gluten-intolerant or coeliac)
1 teaspoon baking powder
3 tablespoons macadamia oil
Guacamole (page 194), to serve (optional)

Blitz the macadamia nuts in a food processor until finely chopped and set aside.

Place half the corn kernels into the bowl of a food processor, along with the onion, eggs and coriander. Add a pinch of salt and pepper and blend until about three-quarters of the corn is puréed. Transfer the mixture to a large bowl and stir through the remaining corn, chopped macadamia nuts, flour and baking powder until just combined. Don't overmix.

Heat 1 tablespoon of the oil in a large shallow frying pan over medium-high heat. When the oil is hot, add heaped tablespoons of the mixture to the pan (you should be able to cook 5 or 6 fritters at a time). Cook for 1–2 minutes each side until golden and just cooked. You can keep the first batch warm in a 100°C (210°F) oven while you cook the rest. Serve the fritters with the guacamole, if desired.

Store in a sealed container in the refrigerator for up to 2 days.

> **For younger babies** purée half a cooked fritter, ½ tablespoon ole (if using) and a tablespoon or two of water until smooth.
>
> **For older babies** mash coarsely. Alternatively the fritters make ideal finger food for babies who can chew their food, but be sure the macadamia nuts are very finely chopped.
>
> **For toddlers** serve as for adults, but ensure that any nuts are finely chopped.

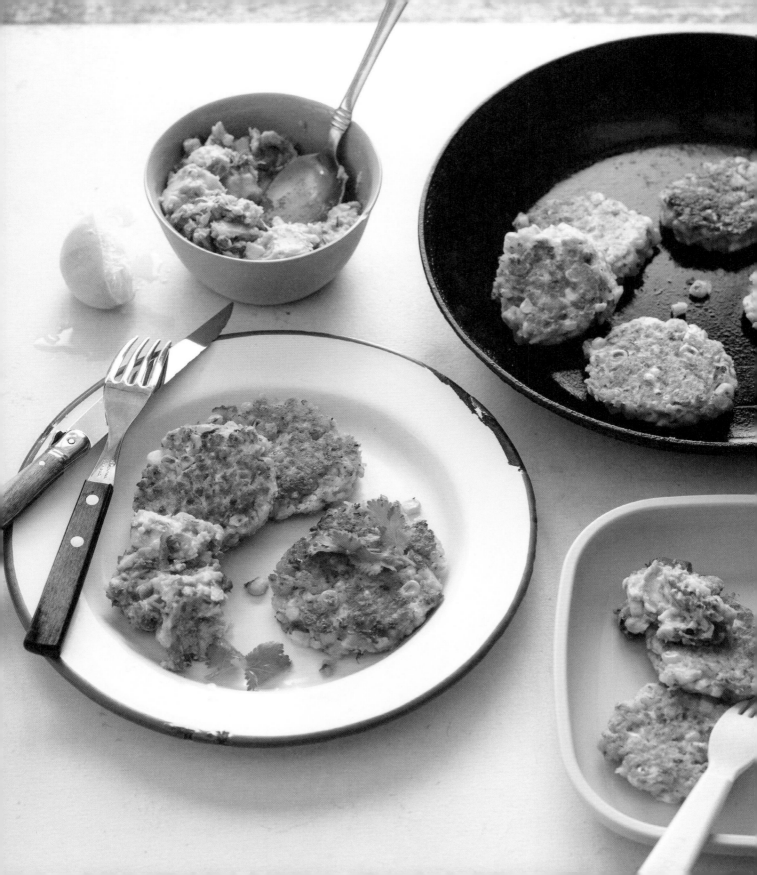

FRENCH TOAST

SERVES 4

PREP TIME: 10 MINUTES

COOKING TIME: 5 MINUTES

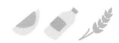

French toast is, in our opinion, best made with brioche as it's rich and buttery, but of course this is also fantastic made with good old-fashioned yesterday's bread – preferably sourdough. We serve the French toast here simply with maple syrup and banana, but for adults you can swap the banana for bacon, or alternately just serve with a good drizzle of Berry purée (see page 188).

4 eggs
250 ml (8¼ fl oz/1 cup) full-cream
   (whole) milk
1 teaspoon natural vanilla extract
4 thick slices of brioche or yesterday's
   bread (preferably sourdough)
50 g (1¾ oz) butter
2 fresh, soft bananas, peeled and
   thickly sliced
maple syrup, to serve
ground cinnamon, to serve
   (just a tiny amount for babies)

Beat the eggs together with the milk and vanilla in a large shallow bowl. Add the brioche/bread slices and let them soak up the egg mixture for a few minutes.

Heat a large non-stick frying pan over high heat and add the butter. When the butter is bubbling, give the brioche/bread slices one final thorough dip in the egg mixture, drain the excess (just lightly as you want all the egg you can get) and add each slice to the pan. You may need to cook the toast in 2 batches. Cook for about 2 minutes on each side until golden and crusty, then transfer the slices to serving plates.

Share the sliced banana across the plates and finish with a drizzle of maple syrup and a sprinkling of cinnamon.

> **For younger babies 7 months plus** French toast is great finger food. Trim the crusts off the bread before adding it to the egg batter to make the French toast softer for baby. Cut the French toast into 'soldiers' (finger-sized pieces).
>
> **For older babies** cut the toast into soldiers and serve with mashed banana.
>
> **For toddlers** cut the toast into soldiers and serve with sliced banana - and a drizzle of maple syrup for older toddlers.

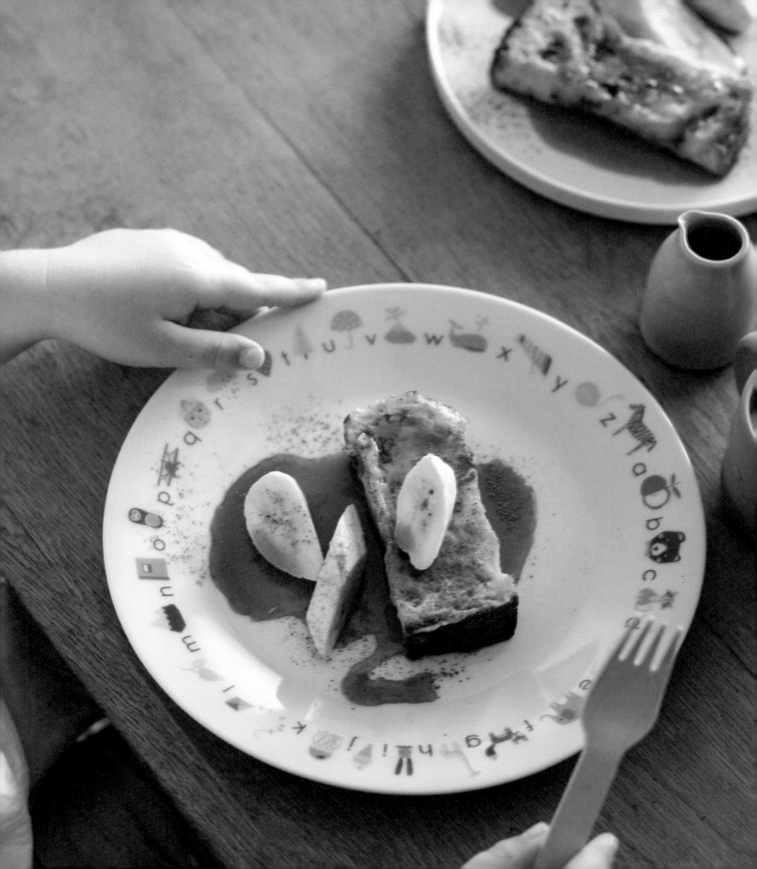

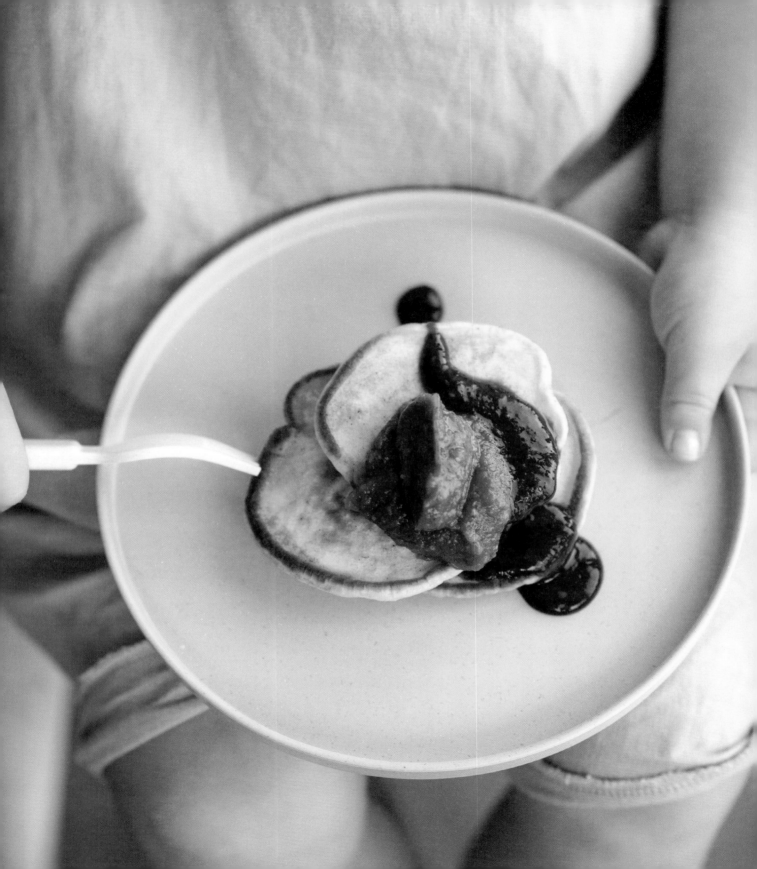

PIKELETS WITH APPLE BUTTER AND BERRIES

SERVES 4 (MAKES 12)

PREP TIME: 5 MINUTES, PLUS RESTING

COOKING TIME: 5 MINUTES

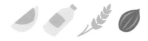

Whether for breakfast, brunch or dessert, these mini pancake-style treats are a family favourite in our house, especially when we are on holiday or celebrating. They are great as they are, but particularly good served with Apple butter with hazelnut, prune and cinnamon, and with Berry purée.

190 ml (6½ fl oz/¾ cup) milk
1 egg
150 g (5½ oz/1 cup) self-raising flour (substitute gluten-free flour if family members are gluten-intolerant or coeliac)
sea salt (omit for babies)
butter, for cooking
Apple butter with hazelnut, prune and cinnamon (page 216), to serve
Berry purée (see page 188), to serve

Whisk the milk and egg together in a mixing bowl. In a separate bowl sift the flour with a pinch of salt.

Add the dry ingredients to the wet and whisk well until smooth. Rest for 15 minutes.

Heat a medium non-stick frying pan over medium heat and add 2 teaspoons butter. When just bubbling, add 1 tablespoon of the batter to the pan and repeat until you have 4 pikelets in the pan. Cook for about 30 seconds or until bubbles appear on the surface. Turn and cook on the other side for 1 minute, or until golden. Remove the pikelets from the pan and set aside while you cook the remainder.

Serve the pikelets warm with the apple butter and a drizzle of berry purée.

Store in a sealed container in the refrigerator for up to 2 days, or freeze in a sealed bag for up to 3 months.

> **For younger babies 7 months plus** these make ideal finger food. Cut the pikelets into soft 'soldiers' (finger-sized pieces) and smear with apple butter - always stay with your baby when they are experimenting with finger foods.
>
> **For older babies** cut the pikelets into soldiers and smear with apple butter and berry purée.
>
> **For toddlers** cut the pikelets into soldiers and let your toddler dip them into the apple butter and berry purée.

soups
and salads

CHINESE-STYLE CHICKEN, SWEET CORN AND EGG SOUP

SERVES 4-6

PREP TIME: 10 MINUTES

COOKING TIME: 20 MINUTES

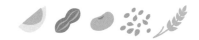

This comforting and delicious soup is full of both protein and vegetables. For the adults, serve with some Asian fried shallots and chilli sauce.

1 litre (34 fl oz/4 cups) quality chicken stock (preferably preservative and additive free)

2 skinless, boneless chicken breasts

kernels from 4 corn cobs (you will need about 400 g/14 oz kernels)

1 tablespoon peanut oil

1 tablespoon grated fresh ginger

1 garlic clove, crushed (just a tiny amount for babies)

2 French shallots, thinly sliced

1 tablespoon cornflour (cornstarch) and 1 tablespoon water

2 teaspoons sesame oil

2 eggs

2 tablespoons light soy sauce (omit for babies)

sea salt (omit for babies)

ground white pepper (just a tiny amount for babies)

Place the stock in a large saucepan over high heat. Bring to the boil, then reduce the heat to medium, add the chicken and simmer for 7-8 minutes, or until the chicken is just cooked. Remove the chicken from the stock, allow to cool a little, then shred the meat finely. Set the chicken and pan of stock aside.

Purée half the corn kernels using a hand-held blender, adding a little stock if the mixture is too thick to purée easily.

Heat the peanut oil in a heavy-based frying pan over high heat. Add the ginger and garlic and stir-fry for 30 seconds, then add the shallot and fry for a further 30 seconds. Transfer the ginger, garlic and shallot mixture, the remaining corn kernels and the puréed corn to the saucepan with the reserved stock. Return the stock to the boil and simmer for 10 minutes.

In a bowl, mix the cornflour and water and stir to a smooth paste. Add 80 ml (2½ fl oz/⅓ cup) of the stock to the cornflour and mix well until smooth, then stir the mixture into the soup. Bring slowly to the boil once again and allow the soup to thicken, for about 2 minutes, stirring constantly. Add the chicken to the soup, as well as the sesame oil.

Whisk the eggs with 1 tablespoon of the stock in a small bowl, then drizzle it into the soup very slowly, from about 15 cm (6 in) above the pot - the egg will cook in fine strings. (Remove baby's serve now.) Add the soy sauce and season to taste as required. Add a pinch of ground white pepper to the top of each serve. Store in an airtight container in the refrigerator for up to 2 days, or freeze for up to 3 months.

> **For younger babies** purée until smooth and allow to cool before serving.
>
> **For older babies** purée to a lumpy texture and allow to cool before serving.
>
> **For toddlers** serve as for adults, but allow to cool before serving.

SUMMER MINESTRONE

SERVES 4

PREP TIME: 10 MINUTES

COOKING TIME: 25 MINUTES

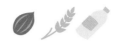

Always a nutritional standout, this 'green' minestrone ticks so many boxes when it comes to food that's healthy, easy and quick to prepare. Make it with best-quality stock and fresh produce and you can't go wrong.

2 tablespoons olive oil

2 tablespoons macadamia oil

1 small brown onion, finely diced

1 leek, white part only, thinly sliced and well washed

4 garlic cloves, finely chopped (just a tiny amount for babies)

2 celery stalks, thinly sliced

2 green zucchini (courgettes), halved lengthways and thinly sliced

1 litre (34 fl oz/4 cups) quality vegetable stock (preferably preservative and additive free) or water

1 bunch asparagus, woody ends snapped off, thinly sliced

100 g (3½ oz/⅔ cup) fresh peas or defrosted frozen peas

200 g (7 oz) green beans, thinly sliced

8 leaves silverbeet (Swiss chard) or rainbow chard, finely shredded

small bunch basil, leaves only

sea salt (omit for babies)

ground white pepper (just a tiny amount for babies)

grated pecorino (use ricotta for babies), to serve

toasted bread, to serve

Place a large saucepan over medium heat and add the oils. Add the onion, leek, garlic and celery and cook gently for 6–8 minutes, or until the vegetables are soft. Add the zucchini and cook for another 2 minutes, then add the stock or water, cover and simmer for 10 minutes. Remove the lid and add the asparagus, peas, beans, silverbeet and basil. Return to the boil, then remove from the heat. Season to taste with salt and pepper. Serve topped with grated pecorino and your favourite toasted bread.

Store in an airtight container in the refrigerator for up to 2 days, or freeze for up to 3 months.

For younger babies purée the soup and ricotta pieces until smooth. For a thicker purée add a small amount of the bread torn up into pieces and purée again. Allow to cool before serving.

For older babies tear some bread into pieces and add it to the soup to soften, before briefly blitzing with a hand-held blender to a lumpy consistency. Allow to cool before serving.

For toddlers serve the cooled soup with toasted buttery bread 'soldiers' (finger-sized pieces).

ZUCCHINI SOUP WITH GRISSINI DIPPERS

SERVES 4-6

PREP TIME: 10 MINUTES

COOKING TIME: 25 MINUTES

OPTIONAL

Zucchini (courgette) is an inexpensive and much underrated vegetable and makes a delicious soup. The grissini dipping sticks make the meal great fun and a perfect finger food for kids. You can further jazz it up by adding a nutty component with a swirl of hazelnut oil before adding the cheese.

3 tablespoons olive oil

50 g (1¾ oz) butter

4 green zucchini (courgettes), thickly sliced into rounds

½ large bunch basil, leaves only

4 garlic cloves, chopped (just a tiny amount for babies)

sea salt (omit for babies)

ground white pepper (just a tiny amount for babies)

125 ml (4 fl oz/½ cup) pouring (single/light) cream

grated pecorino (use ricotta for babies), to serve

grissini or crusty bread, to serve

Place a large saucepan over medium heat and add the olive oil and butter. When the butter has melted, add the zucchini, basil, garlic and a good pinch of salt. Stir well and cook slowly, stirring, for 15 minutes to allow the zucchini to break down a little. The mixture will be fragrant from the basil and garlic. Add enough hot water to just cover (be careful not to add more than this or your soup will be insipid). Return to the boil, then simmer until the zucchini is soft. Add the cream, then purée the mixture using a hand-held blender.

Check the seasoning and adjust. Serve with a little grated pecorino on top and grissini sticks or crusty bread for dipping.

Store in an airtight container in the refrigerator for up to 2 days, or freeze for up to 3 months.

> **For younger babies** add the grissini sticks or bread before puréeing the soup until smooth, to thicken it up. Allow to cool before serving.
>
> **For older babies** serve as is but allow to cool before serving. Make sure the grissini or bread is in small finger-sized pieces, if using.
>
> **For toddlers** serve as for adults, but allow to cool before serving.

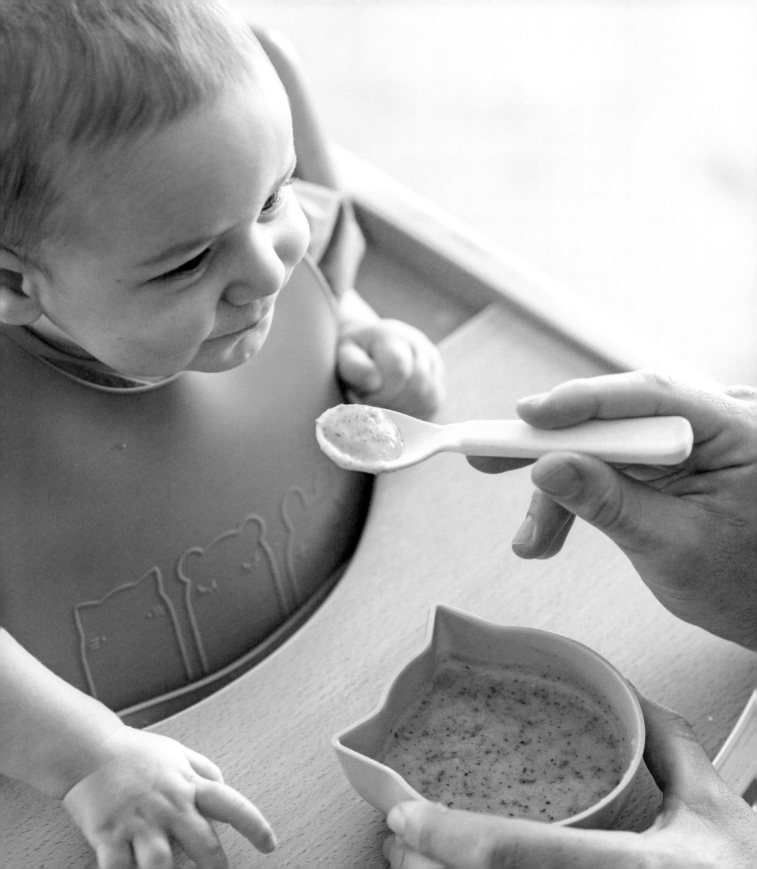

RIBOLLITA

OPTIONAL

This is a heartwarming and nutritious soup. Cavolo nero is pretty much a given if you are adding greens to your ribollita, but curly kale and silverbeet (Swiss chard) are great alternatives. Some cooks add zucchini (courgette), diced prosciutto, leeks, thyme leaves, fennel seeds – and crushed dried chillies for the adults. We like to pour in a spoon of lemon oil at the last minute to brighten up the flavours.

2 tablespoons olive oil, plus extra
    to serve
2 brown onions, roughly chopped
3 carrots, roughly chopped
2 garlic cloves, finely chopped (just
    a tiny amount for babies)
3 celery stalks, roughly chopped
2 large tomatoes, roughly chopped
400 g (14 oz) tinned cannellini beans,
    rinsed and drained
1 litre (34 fl oz/4 cups) quality vegetable
    stock (preferably preservative and
    additive free)
2 bay leaves (fresh or dried)
4 large handfuls of cavolo nero (or
    curly kale or silverbeet/Swiss chard),
    roughly chopped
sea salt (omit for babies)
freshly ground black pepper (just a tiny
    amount for babies)
lemon-infused oil (e.g. infused
    macadamia or olive oil) or grated
    lemon zest, to serve (optional)
sliced ciabatta or similar bread, to
    serve
grated parmesan, to serve (use ricotta
    for babies)

Place a medium-large saucepan over medium-low heat and add the olive oil. Toss in the onion, carrot, garlic and celery and leave to cook, stirring occasionally, for 6–8 minutes, until the vegetables are softened.

Add the tomatoes and their juices, the beans, vegetable stock and bay leaves. Simmer for about 30 minutes to bring the ingredients together.

Add the cavolo nero and stir well. Continue to simmer for 15–20 minutes until the greens are wilted. Transfer to serving bowls and season with salt and pepper. Add a drizzle of lemon-infused oil or a sprinkle of lemon zest, if desired, and serve with the bread and grated parmesan on the side.

Store in an airtight container in the refrigerator for up to 2 days, or freeze for up to 3 months.

For younger babies tear some bread into pieces and use a hand-held blender to purée the combined soup, bread and ricotta to a smooth consistency. Allow to cool before serving.

For older babies tear some bread into pieces and add it to the soup to soften, before briefly blitzing with a hand-held blender to a lumpy consistency. Allow to cool before serving.

For toddlers serve as for adults, but allow to cool before serving.

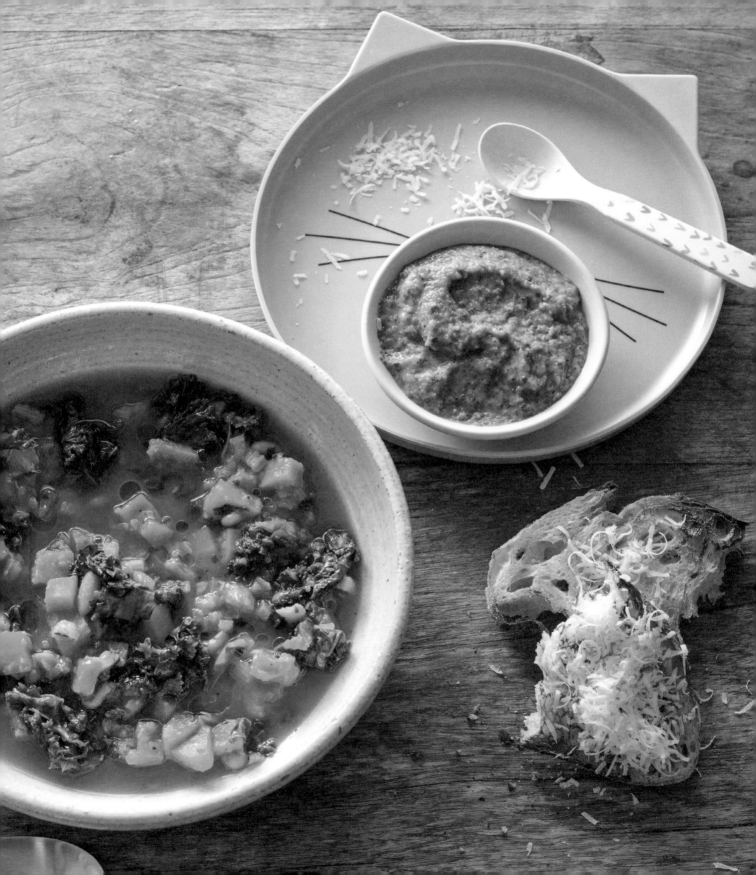

CHICKEN AND GINGER CONGEE

Congee is a soup and a breakfast, lunch or dinner! This light Chinese variation is full-flavoured and nutritious. We love to add a fried or chopped boiled egg, and you can use up last night's rice by adapting this recipe – simply add the rice and chicken to a saucepan and cover with water by a good 4 cm (1½ in). Bring slowly up to heat, add your seasonings, check the consistency and off you go. For adults, kimchi and chilli sauce are the perfect additions.

SERVES 6

PREP TIME: 10 MINUTES

COOKING TIME: 40 MINUTES

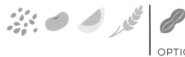

OPTIONAL

500 ml (17 fl oz/2 cups) quality chicken stock (preferably preservative and additive free) mixed with 1 litre (34 fl oz/4 cups) water

2 teaspoons shaoxing rice wine

2 cm (¾ in) piece fresh ginger, cut into thin matchsticks

200 g (7 oz/1 cup) jasmine rice

400 g (14 oz) skinless boneless chicken thighs, diced into 1 cm (½ in) pieces

½ teaspoon sesame oil

3 tablespoons light soy sauce, or to taste (omit for babies)

fried eggs (hard-boiled for babies), to serve

thinly sliced spring onion (scallion), green parts only, to serve

store-bought Asian fried shallots, to serve

coarsely ground white pepper (just a tiny amount for babies)

kimchi, to serve (omit for babies and for toddlers not ready for spice) (check the label for allergens)

chilli sauce, to serve (omit for babies and for toddlers not ready for spice)

Bring the stock and water, rice wine and ginger to the boil in a medium saucepan over high heat. Add the rice and reduce the heat to medium-low. Simmer steadily for 30 minutes, stirring occasionally - to prevent the rice from catching - until it's thickened and most of the liquid has been absorbed. Add the chicken and sesame oil, plus an extra 500 ml (17 fl oz/2 cups) water. Cover and simmer for 4-5 minutes, or until the chicken is just cooked. Check the consistency at this point - it should be more soupy than 'rice'. (Set younger or older baby's serve aside now.) Add the soy sauce and heat through for a minute - add a little more water if necessary and keep checking your seasoning for balance.

Serve the congee in bowls, topped with a fried egg and sprinkled with the sliced spring onion, fried shallots and white pepper. Add a little extra sesame oil or soy, if desired. Add the kimchi and chilli sauce and serve. Store in an airtight container in the refrigerator for up to 2 days, or freeze for up to 3 months.

For younger babies purée using a hand-held blender until smooth. You can also add a dollop of smooth, unsalted peanut butter (see Home-made nut butters on page 217) or some puréed hard-boiled egg. Allow to cool before serving.

For older babies purée the soup to a lumpy consistency and add a dollop of smooth, unsalted peanut butter and some chopped hard-boiled egg. Allow to cool before serving.

For toddlers serve as for adults, but allow to cool before serving.

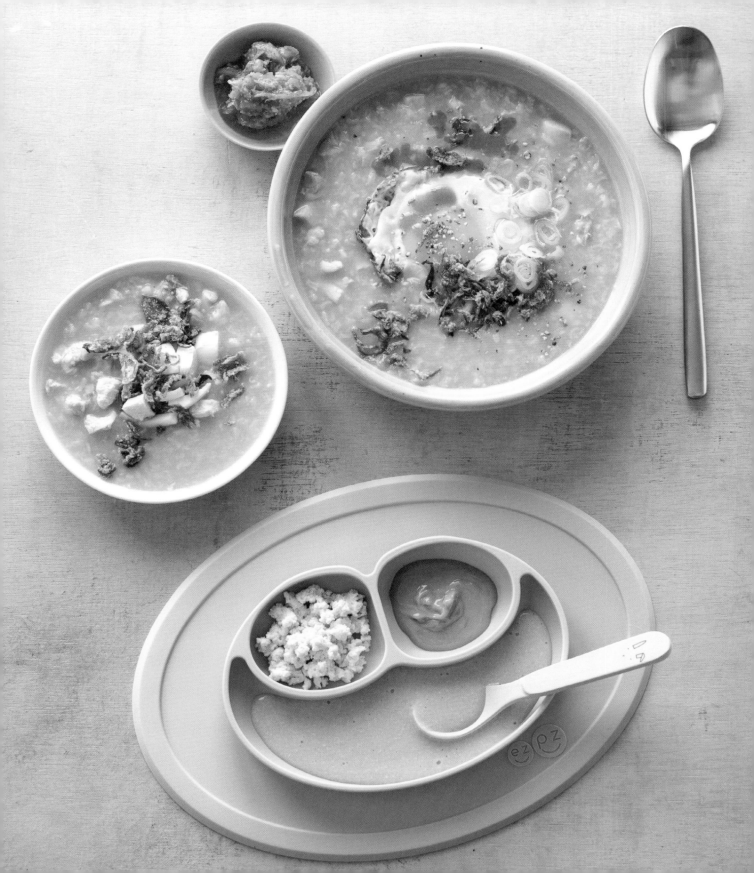

PANZANELLA

SERVES 6

PREP TIME: 10 MINUTES

**COOKING TIME: 5 MINUTES
(40 MINUTES IF ROASTING
YOUR OWN PEPPERS)**

OPTIONAL

This is a traditional Italian bread and tomato salad, great as a side, but hearty enough to serve as a meal on its own. It's a great use for day-old bread.

400 g (14 oz/2 cups) roughly chopped ripe tomatoes, or use a mix of yellow and red cherry tomatoes, halved, for colour
sea salt (omit for babies)
freshly ground black pepper (just a tiny amount for babies)
2 tablespoons baby capers, rinsed and drained
1 small red onion, halved and thinly sliced
200 g (7 oz) store-bought roasted red peppers, drained and roughly torn (see Note)
2 anchovy fillets, thinly sliced (omit for babies)
200 g (7 oz) day-old sourdough bread or ciabatta, roughly torn and dried out in a warm place
2 tablespoons red-wine vinegar
120 ml (4 fl oz) extra virgin olive oil
1 small bunch basil, leaves only

Place the tomatoes in a bowl and season well with salt and pepper. Add the capers, onion, peppers and anchovies (if using). Mix well, then add the bread and toss everything together to combine. Add the vinegar and oil, toss well and check the seasoning and balance, adding extra salt, pepper, vinegar and oil as desired. Then add the basil, mix well and serve.

> **For younger babies** purée until smooth - thin it out with a little water if it's too thick.
>
> **For older babies** blitz briefly until lumpy for great finger food.
>
> **For toddlers** serve as for adults.

NOTE: You can make your own roasted peppers by lightly brushing 2 whole red capsicums (bell peppers) with oil, then roasting them on a baking paper–lined tray in a 200°C (400°F) oven for 40 minutes (turning at 20 minutes) until charred, soft and squishy. Allow to cool, then split open and remove the seeds, rub off the charred skin and tear into pieces.

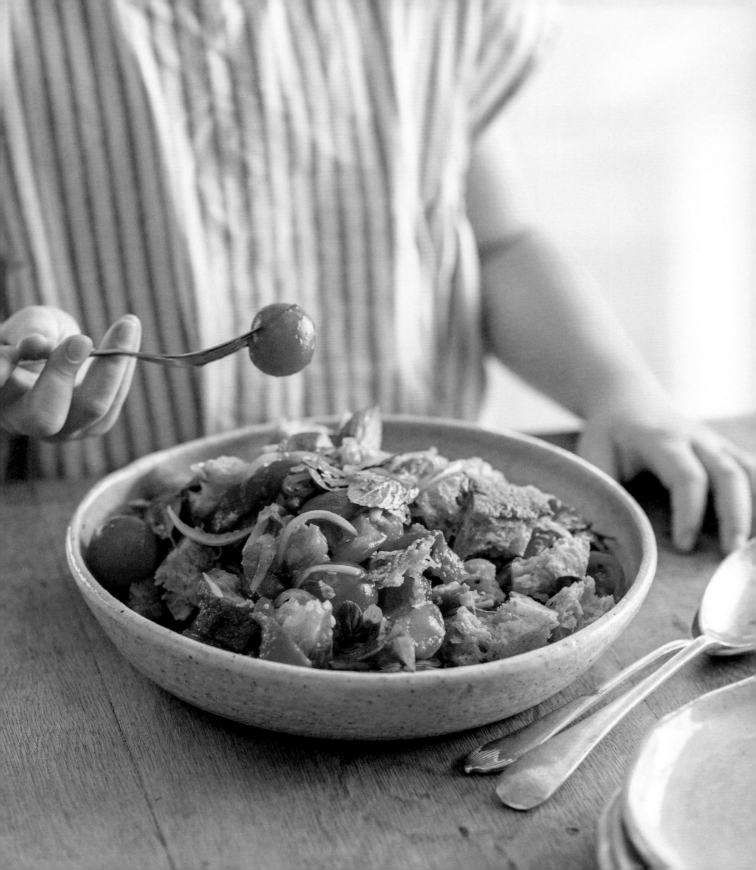

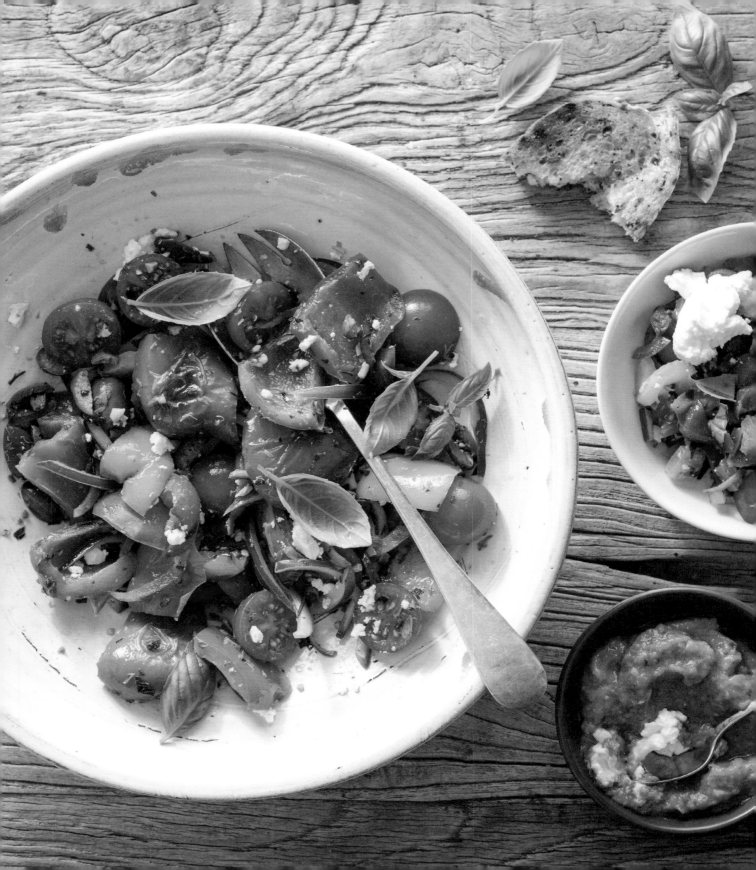

TUSCAN-STYLE SALAD WITH BUFFALO MOZZARELLA

SERVES 4 AS A SIDE

PREP TIME: 15 MINUTES

COOKING TIME: 25 MINUTES

OPTIONAL

You'll find many of the ingredients for this dish in the delicatessen – or maybe even in your refrigerator! The tomatoes and olives make this salad slightly acidic, so serve with rice, polenta or pasta. It is also great served with meat or fish.

1 green capsicum (bell pepper), deseeded and chopped into chunks

1 red capsicum (bell pepper), deseeded and chopped into chunks

1 yellow capsicum (bell pepper), deseeded and chopped into chunks

1 tablespoon macadamia oil

2 garlic cloves, finely chopped (just a tiny amount for babies)

2 oregano sprigs, leaves picked and roughly chopped

360 g (12¼ oz/2 cups) cherry tomatoes, halved

¼ red onion, thinly sliced

90 g (3 oz/¼ cup) green olives, pitted and sliced

2 tablespoons capers, rinsed and drained

2 tablespoons red-wine vinegar

30 g (1 oz/1 loosely packed cup) basil leaves, torn or whole

sea salt (omit for babies)

freshly ground black pepper (just a tiny amount for babies)

1 buffalo mozzarella or 1 tablespoon crumbled feta or shaved pecorino (use ricotta for babies)

olive oil, for drizzling

Preheat the oven to 200°C (400°F). Line a baking tray with baking paper.

In a large mixing bowl, toss the capsicum with the macadamia oil, garlic and oregano.

Transfer to the baking tray and roast for 20-25 minutes. Remove from the oven, cover with foil and allow to cool.

Meanwhile, place the cherry tomatoes in the same large mixing bowl. Add the onion, olives, capers and vinegar. Fold in the basil leaves and season as required.

Transfer to a platter or serving bowl. Tear the buffalo mozzarella on top, drizzle with olive oil and serve.

Store in an airtight container in the refrigerator for up to 24 hours.

> **For younger babies** sprinkle with ricotta to soften the acidity of the tomatoes. Purée until smooth. Add some bread or Baby's first cereal (page 58) to thicken the purée, if desired.
>
> **For older babies** blitz the salad briefly to break down any larger pieces.
>
> **For toddlers** serve as for adults.

POTATO SALAD WITH KING PRAWNS

SERVES 4

PREP TIME: 15 MINUTES

COOKING TIME: 10 MINUTES

A timeless, easy to prepare summer favourite with delicious flavours and textures. You can replace the prawns (shrimp) with salmon or firm white fish fillets, gently cooked and flaked into pieces – but make sure there are no bones!

sea salt
200 g (7 oz) waxy potatoes, such as kipfler (fingerling) or Dutch cream, cut into 1 cm (½ in) dice
160 g (5¼ oz) celeriac, peeled and cut into 1 cm (½ in) dice
2 carrots, cut into 1 cm (½ in) dice
100 g (3½ oz/⅔ cup) frozen peas, defrosted
iced water
3 tablespoons mayonnaise
2 tablespoons crème fraîche or sour cream
1 tablespoon horseradish (omit for babies) (see Notes)
2 tablespoons finely chopped chives
juice of ½ lemon, plus wedges to serve
freshly ground black pepper (just a tiny amount for babies)
8–12 cooked king prawns (jumbo shrimp), peeled and deveined, tails left on, to serve, or 2 x 140 g (5 oz) salmon or firm white fish fillets (see Notes)

Bring a large saucepan of water to the boil over high heat. Add a good pinch of salt, then add the potato, celeriac and carrot. Simmer for 5-7 minutes, adding the peas for the last 30 seconds, until the vegetables are tender but still slightly al dente. Drain well, then immediately immerse the vegetables in a bowl of iced water to refresh, for about 1 minute - this retains the colour of the vegies. Drain well.

In a large bowl, combine the mayonnaise, crème fraîche, horseradish, chives and lemon juice. Add the cooled vegetables, toss to coat and season to taste with salt and pepper. Serve with the prawns and lemon wedges.

> **For younger babies** chop 1 small prawn, tail removed (or some cooked flaked fish with no bones) . Add the coated salad vegies, a squeeze of lemon juice and a tablespoon of water to thin it, then purée until smooth.
>
> **For older babies** chop 1 small prawn, tail removed (or some cooked flaked fish with no bones). Add the coated salad vegies, then blitz briefly with a squeeze of lemon juice until you have a lumpy texture.
>
> **For toddlers** serve as for adults.

NOTES: If in season you could replace the store-bought horseradish with some horseradish root freshly grated over the top of the salad just before serving. If using fish instead of prawns, fry the fillet gently with a couple of tablespoons of olive oil in a frying pan for 3 minutes each side. Allow to cool, then remove the skin and flake the flesh. Ensure there are no bones.

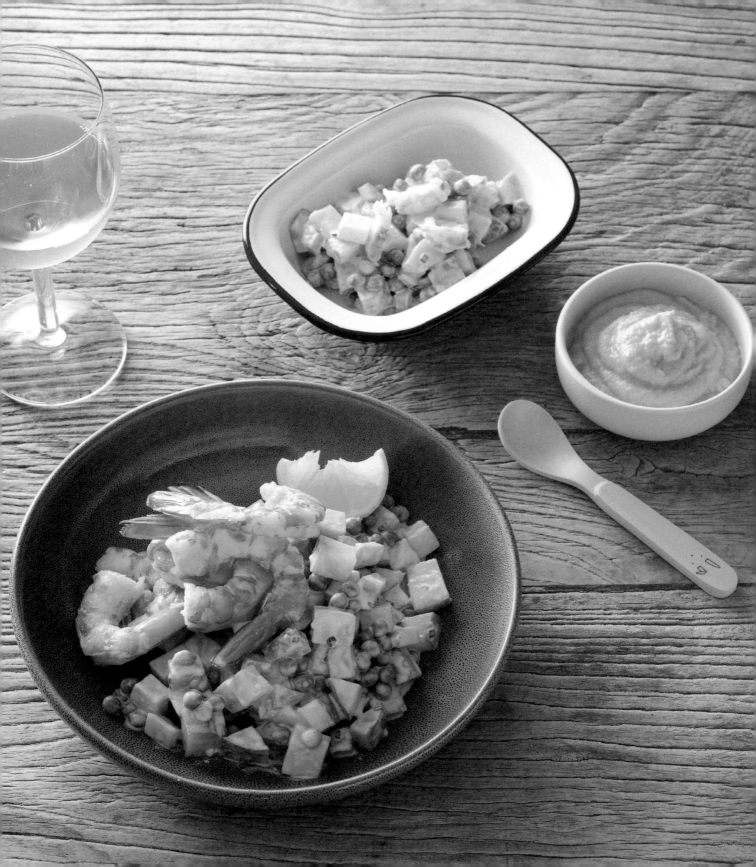

FRAGRANT THAI-STYLE BEEF SALAD

SERVES 4

PREP TIME: 15 MINUTES

COOKING TIME: 12 MINUTES

OPTIONAL

This is a fresh and fragrant salad with a hint of punch and crunch, and it's packed full of protein. Leftovers can be reheated the next day or added to Bubble and squeak (page 74).

2 tablespoons macadamia or other nut oil
2 garlic cloves, crushed (just a tiny amount for babies)
1 teaspoon minced fresh ginger
500 g (1 lb 2 oz) lean minced (ground) beef
150 g (5½ oz) green beans, trimmed and sliced into 1 cm (½ in) pieces
1 lemongrass stem, white part only, finely chopped
40 g (1½ oz/¼ cup) peanuts, skin on, finely chopped (optional – you can use tree nuts as an alternative)
150 g (5½ oz/2 cups) finely shredded Chinese cabbage (wombok)
finely grated zest and juice of 1 lime, plus wedges to serve
pinch of caster (superfine) sugar
1 long red chilli, deseeded and thinly sliced (omit for babies)
1 tablespoon fish sauce (omit for babies)
4 spring onions (scallions), thinly sliced
small handful of coriander (cilantro), leaves roughly chopped
small handful of mint leaves, roughly chopped
8 butter lettuce leaf cups, to serve

Heat a wok over high heat and add the oil. Stir-fry the garlic and ginger quickly to caramelise, then add the beef. Toss well and brown the meat for 5 minutes, stirring to break up any lumps. Add the beans, lemongrass and peanuts and stir-fry for 3 minutes. Add the cabbage, lime zest and juice, and sugar. Mix the ingredients through and cook for 2 minutes until the cabbage softens a little. (Remove baby's serve now.)

Add the chilli to the wok and cook for another 2 minutes, then add the fish sauce and stir through for another minute. Remove the wok from the heat, add the spring onion and herbs and toss to combine.

To serve, fill the lettuce leaf cups with the cooked beef mixture and serve with lime wedges on the side to squeeze over.

> **For younger babies** purée a lettuce leaf with 2 tablespoons beef mixture (no spice as per omissions), a few mint and coriander leaves and 2–3 tablespoons water.
>
> **For older babies** sprinkle baby's serve with mint and coriander leaves – this makes great finger food.
>
> **For toddlers** serve as for adults.

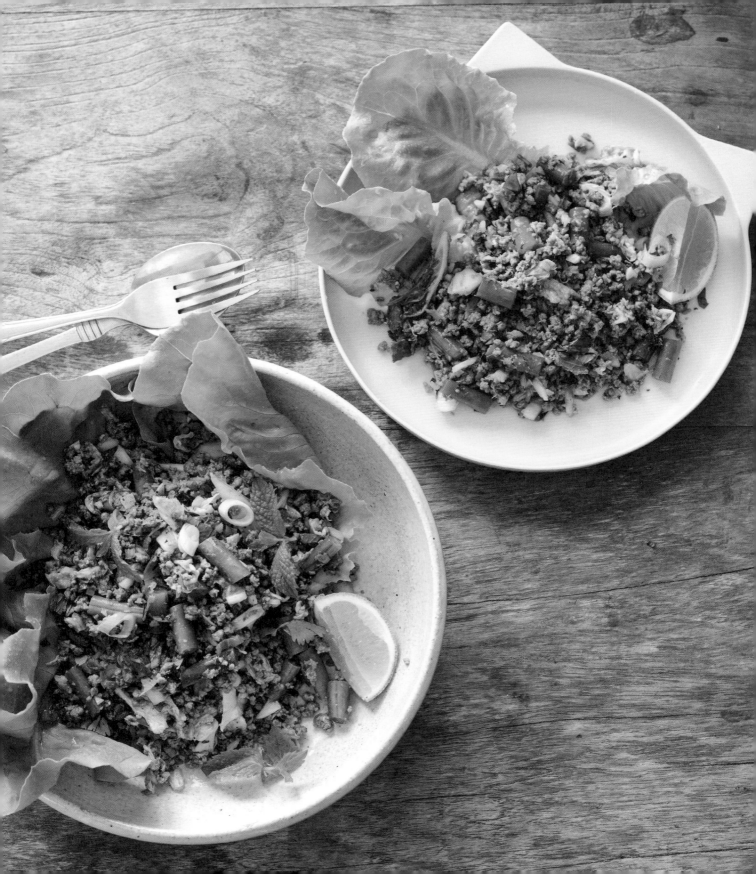

rice,
polenta
and pasta

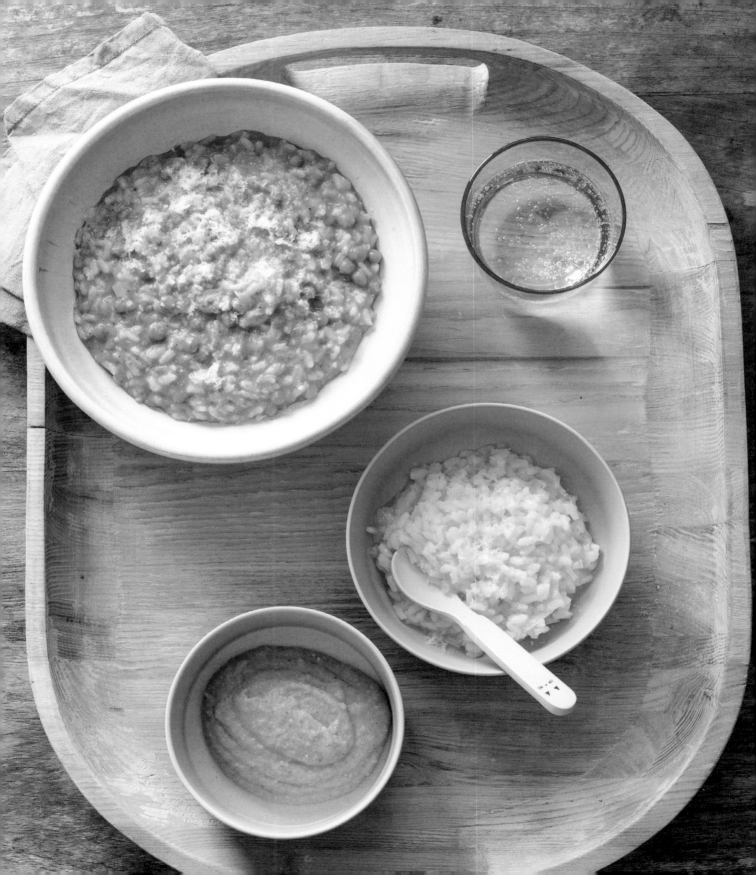

BASIC RISOTTO

SERVES 4

PREP TIME: 5 MINUTES

COOKING TIME: 20 MINUTES

This risotto takes only 20 minutes to cook properly, but it needs your constant attention for the stirring. Once you have mastered the simple art of making risotto, the flavour options are many and varied. Feel free to swap the white wine for red wine and serve it simply as is, with some grated pecorino. Carnaroli is the best risotto rice, but you can also use arborio.

1–2 litres (34–68 fl oz/4–8 cups) quality vegetable or chicken stock (preferably preservative and additive free)
3 tablespoons olive oil
1 brown onion, finely diced
2 garlic cloves, crushed (just a tiny amount for babies)
sea salt (omit for babies)
240 g (8½ oz/1 cup) carnaroli rice
150 ml (5 fl oz) white wine
freshly ground black pepper (just a tiny amount for babies)
grated pecorino, to serve

Bring the stock to the boil in a saucepan and set aside on a very low heat.

Place a medium heavy-based saucepan over medium heat and add the olive oil. Add the onion and garlic with a pinch of salt and sweat until soft, about 5 minutes. Add the rice and stir through for 1 minute to coat well. Add the wine, stir it through and allow the alcohol to cook off and the liquid to be absorbed, then begin to add the stock in small amounts, about a cup at a time, stirring it through and letting it be completely absorbed by the rice before adding the next amount. Continue the process, stirring regularly, until all the stock is absorbed and the rice is tender but not soft. Check the seasoning and adjust as necessary. Serve immediately with grated pecorino.

Store in an airtight container in the refrigerator for up to 2 days, or freeze for up to 3 months.

> **For younger babies** purée the risotto until smooth - thin with a little water if necessary. Use just a touch of finely grated pecorino. Allow to cool before serving.
>
> **For older babies** serve with just a touch of finely grated pecorino. Allow to cool before serving.
>
> **For toddlers** serve as for adults, but allow to cool before serving.

>

Variations

The great thing about risotto is that you can add your choice of proteins and flavours to your base recipe. For the most part, these can be cooked separately and folded through later.

GREEN RISOTTO

Make your risotto as per the basic recipe on page 107. Add 125 g (4½ oz) defrosted frozen peas to a food processor along with 2 large handfuls of baby English spinach leaves and a dash of olive oil. Purée until smooth. Add the pea and spinach purée and a further 125 g (4½ oz) peas to the risotto and stir through. Heat through for 3 minutes, adding a little more stock to keep the risotto soupy. (Set aside baby's portion now.) Season to taste, then add a little grated parmesan and 2 tablespoons chopped flat-leaf (Italian) or curly parsley. Store in an airtight container in the refrigerator for up to 2 days, or freeze for up to 3 months.

> **For younger babies** purée until smooth – thin with a little water if necessary. Allow to cool before serving.
>
> **For older babies** serve with just a touch of finely grated parmesan. Allow to cool before serving.
>
> **For toddlers** serve as for adults, but allow to cool before serving.

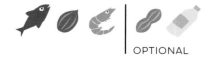

OPTIONAL

SEAFOOD AND CAULIFLOWER RISOTTO

Make your risotto as per the basic recipe on page 107. At the end, add 140 g (5 oz) cooked, flaked boneless white fish or salmon, and ½ cauliflower that has been broken into florets and roasted or pan-fried in a little macadamia oil until crispy. Heat through for 3 minutes, adding a little more stock to keep the risotto soupy. Season to taste and serve topped with your favourite nut or prawn (shrimp) oil. Store in an airtight container in the refrigerator for up to 2 days, or freeze for up to 3 months.

> **For younger babies** purée until smooth – thin with a little water if necessary. Allow to cool before serving.
>
> **For older babies** serve with just a touch of finely grated pecorino. Allow to cool before serving.
>
> **For toddlers** serve as for adults, but allow to cool before serving.

PILAF

SERVES 4

PREP TIME: 3 MINUTES

COOKING TIME: 30 MINUTES

Pilaf is simple yet filling and can be prepped and cooked in just over 30 minutes. Serve it with Lamb meatballs with minted yoghurt sauce (page 167) or Gentle Indian curry of pumpkin and green lentils (page 131.)

40 g (1½ oz) ghee
1 brown onion, finely chopped
1 garlic clove, crushed (just a tiny
   amount for babies)
½ teaspoon cardamom seeds, crushed
1 cinnamon stick, broken in half
3 bay leaves
300 g (10½ oz/1½ cups) basmati rice,
   rinsed
650 ml (22 fl oz) quality chicken stock
   (preferably preservative and
   additive free)
tiny pinch of sea salt (omit for babies)

Heat the ghee in a medium saucepan over low heat. Add the onion and garlic and sweat for 5 minutes or until soft. Add the spices and bay leaves and cook, stirring occasionally, for about 3 minutes or until aromatic. Increase the heat a little. Add the rice and cook, stirring regularly, for about 2 minutes or until coated with ghee and lightly toasted. Add the stock and the salt and stir. Increase the heat to high and bring to the boil. Once boiling, reduce the heat to low again, cover and simmer for 15 minutes, or until all the liquid has been absorbed.

Remove from the heat and allow to rest, covered, for 5 minutes. This gives the rice time to absorb any further liquid.

Store in an airtight container in the refrigerator for up to 2 days.

> **For younger babies** purée the pilaf until smooth - thin with a little water if necessary. Serve with a vegie purée. Allow to cool before serving.
>
> **For older babies and toddlers** serve as for adults, but allow to cool before serving. This is great toddler finger food, but also perfect for learning how to use a spoon.

MILD SALMON KEDGEREE

SERVES 2

PREP TIME: 5 MINUTES

COOKING TIME: 20-25 MINUTES

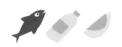

This Indian dish is a warming one-pot winner that can transition into Bubble and squeak (page 74) the next day. Feel free to replace the salmon with boneless white fish fillets. Instead of a hard-boiled egg, a soft-boiled egg can be served to older children and adults.

100 g (3¼ oz/½ cup) basmati rice

2 eggs

20 g (¾ oz) ghee or butter

2 x 100 g (3½ oz) salmon fillets, pin-boned and skin removed

1 garlic clove, finely chopped (just a tiny amount for babies)

1 small brown onion, finely chopped

1 teaspoon finely grated fresh ginger

1 teaspoon curry powder (for babies under 12 months use a mild curry powder or omit)

50 g (1¾ oz) baby English spinach, washed and dried

small handful of finely chopped flat-leaf (Italian) parsley

sea salt (omit for babies)

freshly ground black pepper (just a tiny amount for babies)

lime wedges, to serve

Cook the rice in 250 ml (8½ fl oz/1 cup) water, covered, on very low heat until the water is absorbed and the rice is cooked - this is known as the absorption method. Remove the saucepan from the heat, then lift the lid, cover the pan with a folded tea towel (dish towel) and replace the lid to allow any final steam to absorb.

Boil the eggs for 7 minutes, then cool, peel and quarter them, and set aside. (Ensure the eggs are well cooked if serving to babies.)

In a large frying pan, heat the ghee over medium-high heat. Add the salmon and cook for 3 minutes each side, or until cooked to your liking. Remove the fish from the pan and set aside.

In the same pan over medium heat, sauté the garlic, onion and ginger in the residual ghee for about 7 minutes, until translucent. Reduce the heat, add the curry powder and stir well to combine without letting the ingredients stick to the pan. Add the rice, spinach and parsley. Stir and heat through for 2-3 minutes.

Using a fork, flake the cooked salmon and fold it through the warm rice. Season as required. Transfer to serving plates or a platter and serve with the egg and lime wedges.

Store in an airtight container in the refrigerator for up to 2 days.

NOTE: Always store cooked rice below 4°C (40°F) and reheat until above 60°C (140°F) to ensure there is no trace of *Bacillus cereus*, a harmful bacterial spore that can cause gastric upset. It's best to use cooked rice within 48 hours.

For younger babies purée with egg until smooth - thin with a little water or milk if necessary.

For older babies, if your baby is ready for finger food, coarsely chop the fish and egg and serve as is.

For toddlers serve as for adults.

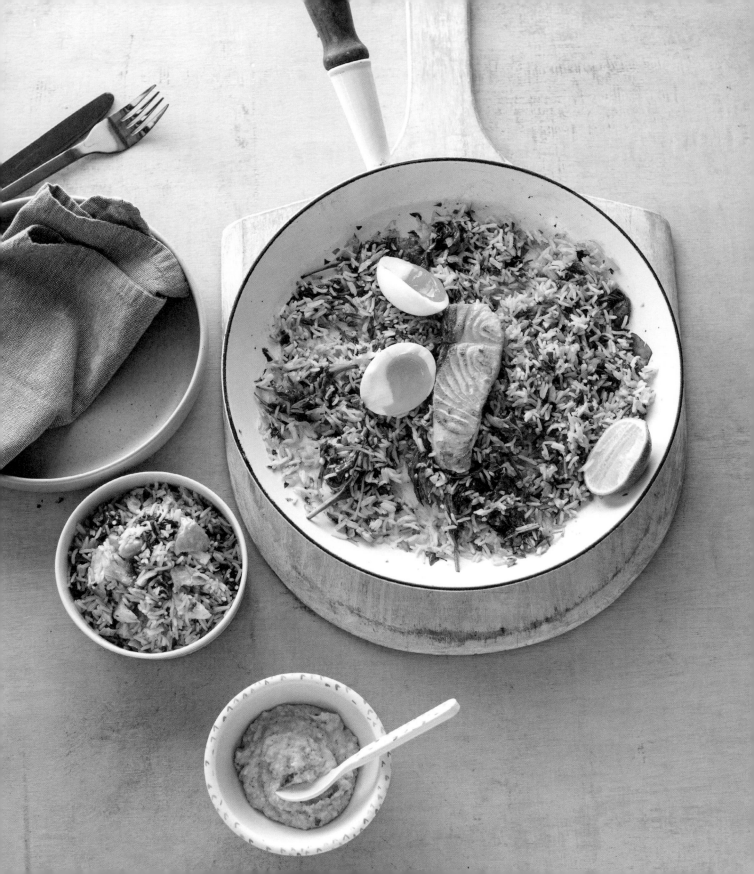

BASIC SOFT POLENTA

SERVES 4

PREP TIME: 5 MINUTES

COOKING TIME: INSTANT POLENTA IS READY IN 5 MINUTES, TRADITIONAL TAKES APPROX. 35 MINUTES

Soft polenta is a blank canvas for some for the most delicious add-ons. It's perfect with Wilted leafy greens with anchovies (page 136), Lamb meatballs with minted yoghurt sauce (page 167), Comforting pork ragu (page 118), or try roasted mushrooms with your favourite herbs – get creative!

400 ml (13¼ fl oz) milk
sea salt
100 g (3½ oz/⅔ cup) polenta (see Note)
40 g (1½ oz) butter
50 g (1¾ oz/½ cup) grated or shaved parmesan (use ricotta for babies)
ground white pepper (just a tiny amount for babies)

Place a medium-sized, wide saucepan over medium heat and add 200 ml (7 fl oz) water and the milk with a pinch of salt. Bring it just to the boil, then slowly and steadily rain in the polenta, whisking constantly. The polenta will return to the boil (watch out for hot exploding bubbles!), at which point turn the heat down as low as you can and cook for about 30 minutes, whisking regularly to avoid any lumps forming. When the polenta is coming away from the edge of the pan, taste it to ensure it is no longer grainy, and that it is cooked. (If using instant polenta, follow the cooking instructions on the packet.) Remove baby's portion now.

Stir through the butter and parmesan. Season with a little more salt, if required (for adults), and some white pepper.

To serve, spoon the polenta generously onto a plate and top with the add-ons of your choice.

Store in an airtight container in the refrigerator for up to 2 days.

> **For younger babies** serve the polenta with some ricotta, but allow it to cool before serving.
>
> **For older babies** serve with wilted greens or mashed meatballs. Allow to cool before serving.
>
> **For toddlers** serve as for adults, but allow to cool before serving.

NOTE: Polenta is coarsely ground cornmeal. Make sure you choose a quality polenta that is GMO free.

GREEN POLENTA

To take your polenta to the next level, blend a mix of finely chopped kale and English or baby spinach leaves (1 handful) with 1 minced garlic clove (just a tiny amount for babies) and 1-2 tablespoons boiling water and stir though the polenta with the butter and parmesan. Store in an airtight container in the refrigerator for up to 2 days.

> **For younger babies** purée until smooth and allow to cool before serving.
>
> **For older babies** serve as is and allow to cool before serving.
>
> **For toddlers** serve as for adults, but allow to cool before serving.

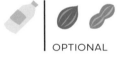

OPTIONAL

BAKED POLENTA

Brush a baking tray (about 16 x 26 cm/6¼ x 10¼ in) with a lip lightly with olive oil or nut oil and line the base and sides with baking paper. Pour in the cooked polenta (as per the basic soft polenta recipe opposite), set aside for 30 minutes to cool, then cover and allow to set in the refrigerator for a minimum of 4 hours or preferably overnight. Preheat the oven to 200°C (400°F). Remove the set polenta from the tray and cut it into squares of approximately 5 cm (2 in). Return to the baking tray, drizzle over a little olive oil and sprinkle with grated parmesan (omit for babies). Bake for 15-20 minutes or until puffed and golden. Store in an airtight container in the refrigerator for up to 2 days.

> **For younger babies** stay with the original softer polenta. Allow to cool before serving.
>
> **For older babies** this makes perfect finger food. Serve as is but allow to cool before serving.
>
> **For toddlers** serve as for adults, but allow to cool before serving.

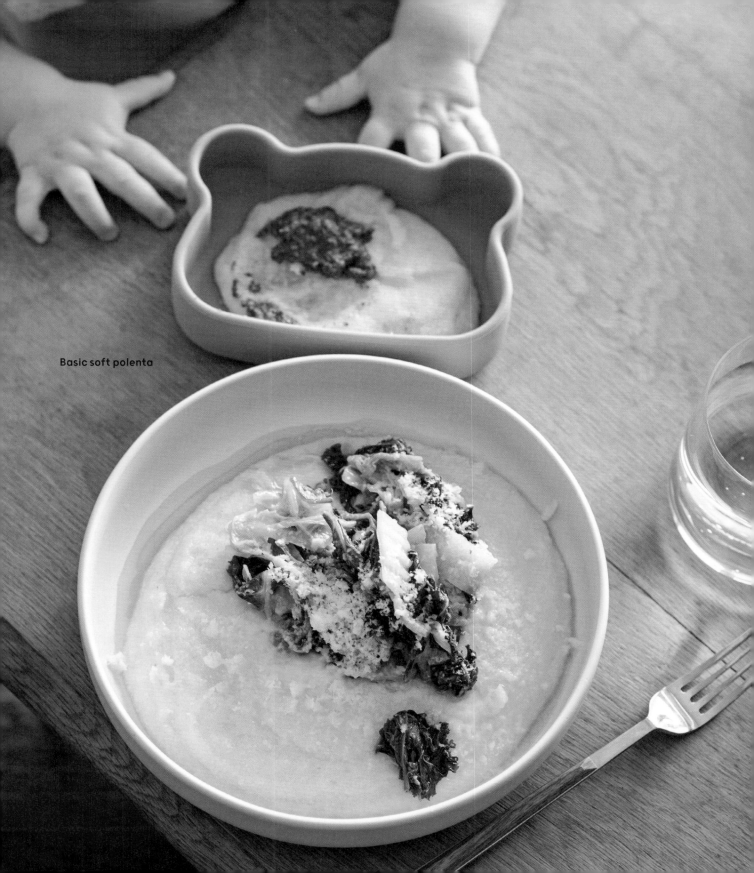

Basic soft polenta

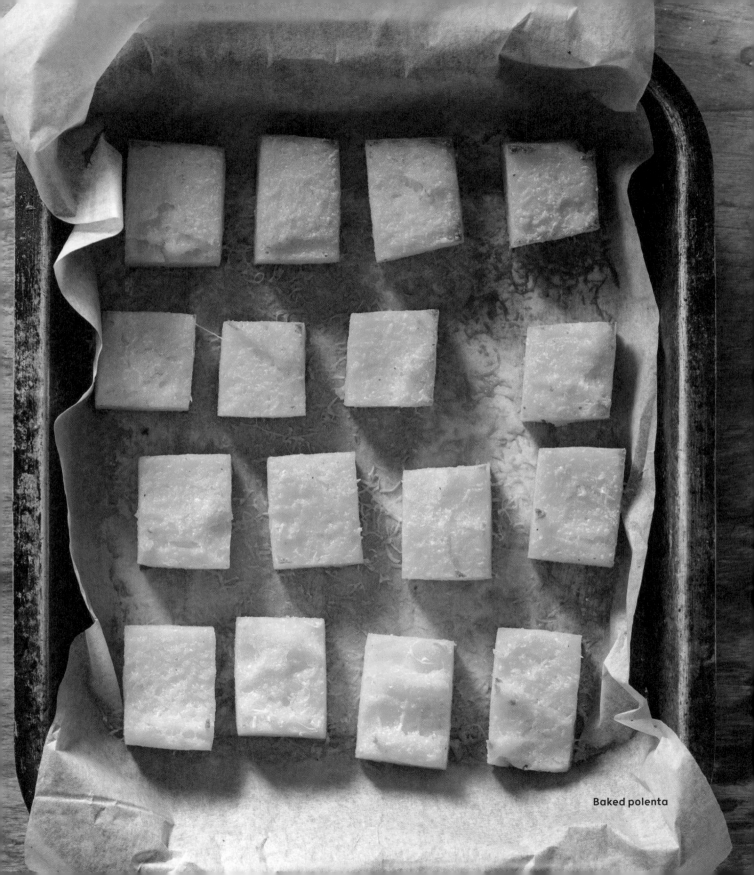

Baked polenta

BASIC POTATO GNOCCHI

SERVES 4

PREP TIME: 15 MINUTES

COOKING TIME: 45 MINUTES

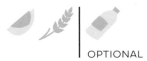

OPTIONAL

Gnocchi is the perfect base for so many toppings. Simply drizzle with olive oil and top with pecorino and fresh herbs. Gnocchi with ragu is a match made in heaven – see Comforting pork ragu (page 118).

8 medium high-starch potatoes
   (Yukon Gold or Desiree potatoes
   are good options)
sea salt (omit for babies)
freshly ground black pepper (just a tiny
   amount for babies)
2 eggs, whisked
plain (all-purpose) flour, to dust
   (substitute with gluten-free flour
   if family members are gluten-
   intolerant or coeliac)

Add the potatoes to a saucepan of cold, salted water and bring to the boil over high heat. When boiling, reduce the heat to medium and cook the potatoes for 20-25 minutes, or until you can easily pierce them with a fork. Drain, then set aside until cool enough to handle but still warm. Using your fingers, remove the skin from the potatoes.

In a medium bowl, mash the warm potatoes until all the lumps are gone. Add salt and pepper, mix well, then make a well in the centre of the potato and add the beaten eggs. Using your hands, gently mix the egg into the potatoes until evenly distributed. Put a little flour onto a clean work surface and turn the potato dough out onto it. Working quickly, knead the dough until it forms a solid round, using as little flour as possible (see Note). Cut the dough into 8 pieces, then roll each piece into a long cylinder about 2 cm (¾ in) thick. Cut the cylinders into 1.5-2 cm (½-¾ in) long pieces and set the pieces of gnocchi aside on a floured board or plate.

Bring a large saucepan of well-salted water to the boil over high heat. Add the gnocchi in small batches, stirring occasionally and gently to ensure they don't stick. Remove them with a slotted spoon or sieve as they rise to the top, about 20-30 seconds. Store in an airtight container in the refrigerator for up to 2 days.

NOTE: When making the gnocchi dough, the potatoes need to be worked quite quickly while warm so as not to overwork the gluten and turn them into rubbery balls.

For younger babies purée with a little water or milk, until smooth and allow to cool before serving.

For older babies this is perfect finger food. Serve the gnocchi with a ladleful of ragu, or just some fresh ricotta and finely chopped herbs. Allow to cool before serving.

For toddlers serve as for adults, but allow to cool before serving.

HOW TO COOK PASTA

OPTIONAL

Pasta comes in all shapes and sizes. Choose a quality durum wheat pasta if you can. There are some excellent gluten-free pastas available in supermarkets too.

Wide, flat pappardelle is great for creamy sauces, and tubular penne is great as a base for meat sauces (see Comforting pork ragu on page 118), as the thick sauce coats the pasta throughout.

350 g (12¼ oz) pasta of your choice
salt

If you are cooking store-bought pasta, you can follow the instructions on the packet. However, here's the way we cook it.

Bring a medium-large saucepan of water to the boil. Add a liberal pinch of salt - this enhances the flavour of the pasta and helps it cook correctly. Add the pasta and stir to separate it, return the water to the boil, then reduce the heat to medium so that it is still ticking over but not on a rapid boil. Stir the pasta occasionally to stop it from sticking to the bottom of the pan and use tongs to separate the strands if cooking long pasta. Cook until al dente - still slightly firm in the centre. Drain the pasta in a colander (see Note), then add your sauce and serve.

> **For younger babies** purée the cooked pasta with the sauce of your choice until smooth (try Comforting pork ragu on page 118 or a vegetable purée with a dollop of ricotta) - you may need to thin it with a little water. Allow to cool before serving.
>
> **For older babies** this makes perfect finger food. Serve with a ladleful of ragu, or with pieces of fresh ricotta and some finely chopped herbs. Allow to cool before serving.
>
> **For toddlers** use alphabet-shaped pasta if you can find it. Toddlers will also enjoy sucking on long spaghetti strings. Allow to cool before serving.

NOTE: Reserve a tablespoon or two of cooking water before draining to add flavour to, and thicken, sauces.

COMFORTING PORK RAGU

SERVES 8

PREP TIME: 7 MINUTES

COOKING TIME: 45 MINUTES

This is family comfort food at its best. The cream soothes the acidity of the tomatoes and beautifully softens this dish. The ragu is delicious served with pasta, gnocchi or polenta.

120 ml (4 fl oz) olive oil

1 brown onion, finely diced

2 garlic cloves, crushed (just a tiny amount for babies)

2 carrots, finely diced

2 celery stalks, finely diced

2 teaspoons finely chopped thyme leaves

½ teaspoon chilli flakes (omit for babies)

500 g (1 lb 2 oz/2¼ cups) chopped tomatoes (or 800 g/1 lb 12 oz tinned chopped tomatoes)

600 g (1 lb 5 oz) minced (ground) pork (or use lamb or beef instead)

500 ml (17 fl oz/2 cups) quality chicken or vegetable stock (preferably preservative and additive free)

150 ml (5 fl oz) pouring (single/light) cream

grated zest of 1 lemon

sea salt (omit for babies)

freshly ground black pepper (just a tiny amount for babies)

cooked pasta, to serve

grated pecorino (use ricotta for babies), to serve

Heat half the oil in a large saucepan over medium heat. Fry the onion and garlic for 4 minutes until soft and caramelised. Add the carrot, celery, thyme and chilli and cook for another 4 minutes. Add the tomatoes and simmer for 15 minutes.

Heat the remaining oil in a medium frying pan over high heat. Add the pork and fry, breaking it up with a wooden spoon, until golden and cooked through, about 8 minutes. Add it to the pan with the vegetable mixture, along with the stock, and simmer over very low heat for 30 minutes.

Add the cream and lemon zest and simmer for a further 5 minutes. Season with salt and pepper to taste. Serve over the cooked pasta of your choice and top with a good sprinkling of grated pecorino (or ricotta for babies).

Store in an airtight container in the refrigerator for up to 2 days, or freeze for up to 3 months.

> **For younger babies** purée the cooked pasta with a little ragu until smooth – you may need to thin it with a little water. Allow to cool before serving.
>
> **For older babies** serve a small amount of coarsely puréed ragu with some pasta. Allow to cool before serving.
>
> **For toddlers** serve as for adults, but allow to cool before serving.

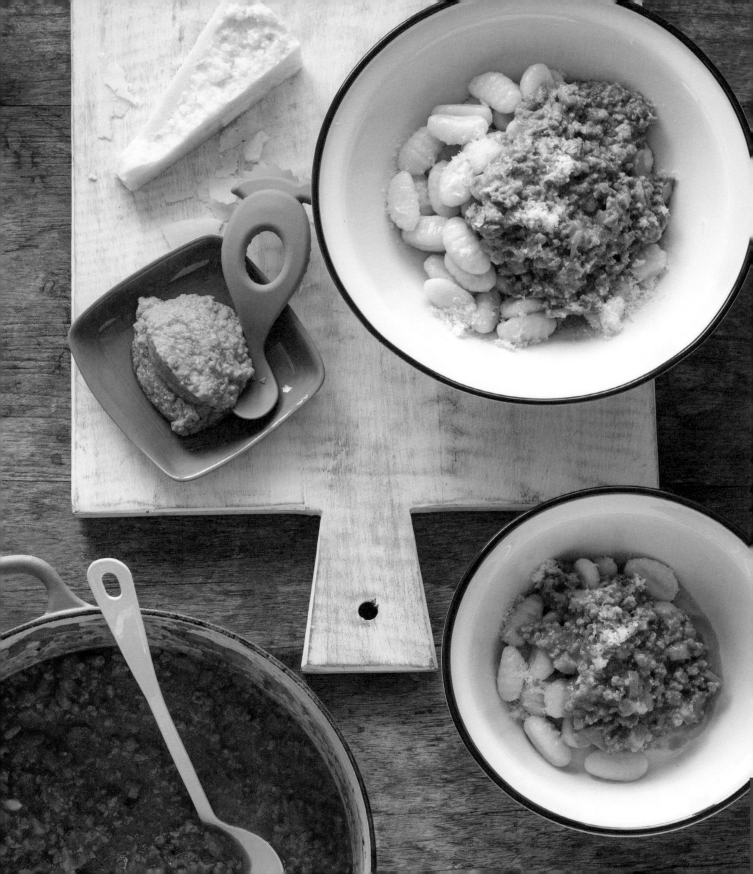

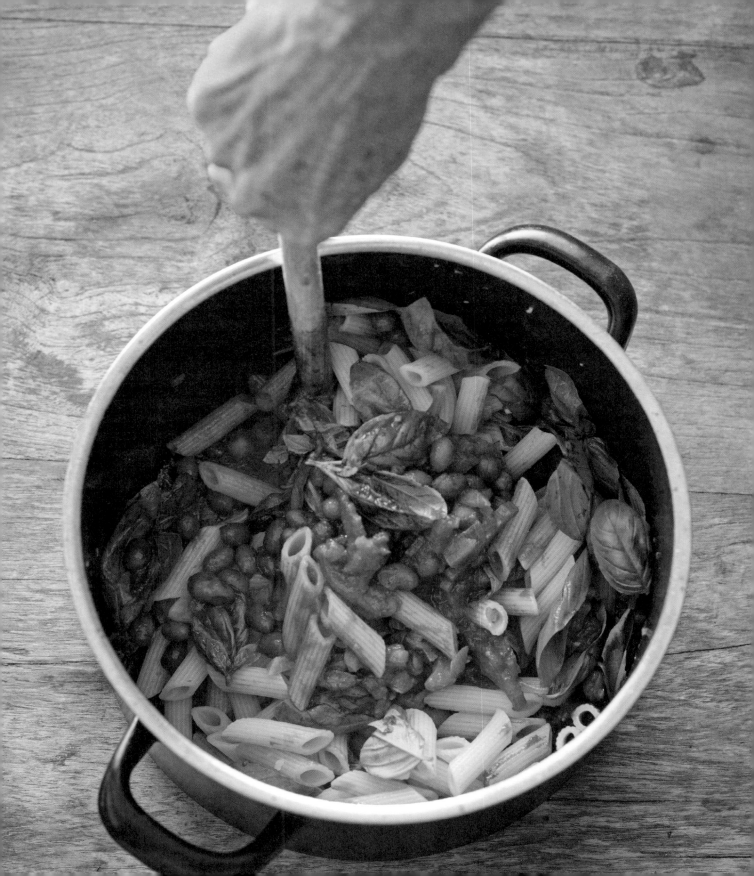

PASTA AND BORLOTTI BEANS

SERVES 4-6

PREP TIME: 5 MINUTES, PLUS OVERNIGHT SOAKING

COOKING TIME: 15 MINUTES

This dish is almost a stew with its large amount of beans among the pasta and tasty sauce. It's a hearty, filling dish that requires nothing more than a green salad to go with it – oh, and perhaps bread for mopping. A delicious high-fibre dinner.

200 g (7 oz/1 cup) dried borlotti (cranberry) beans, soaked overnight (or 400 g/14 oz tinned borlotti beans, rinsed and drained)

2 tablespoons olive oil

1 brown onion, finely diced

1 garlic clove, crushed (just a tiny amount for babies)

1 celery stalk, thinly sliced

30 g (1 oz/1 loosely packed cup) basil leaves

375 g (13 oz/1¼ cups) passata (see Note)

sea salt (omit for babies)

freshly ground black pepper (just a tiny amount for babies)

250 g (9 oz) pasta (small tube shapes such as penne or macaroni are best)

shaved parmesan (use ricotta for babies), to serve

If using soaked dried beans, heat a small saucepan of water over high heat. When boiling, add the drained beans, reduce the heat to low and simmer until soft, about 15 minutes. If using tinned beans, skip this first step.

Meanwhile, place a medium saucepan over medium heat and add the olive oil, followed by the onion and garlic, and cook for 3 minutes until soft and golden. Add the celery, basil, passata and 125 ml (4 fl oz/½ cup) water and bring to the boil, then reduce the heat to low and cook for 5 minutes until it's a little reduced. Add the beans and season with salt and pepper to taste.

Cook the pasta until al dente, then drain and add to the sauce. Stir to combine and heat through. Top with the parmesan to serve.

Store in an airtight container in the refrigerator for up to 2 days.

For younger babies thin with a little water, then purée with some ricotta until smooth. Allow to cool before serving.

For older babies you can coarsely purée the dish, or it makes great finger food. Top with pieces of ricotta. Allow to cool before serving.

For toddlers serve as for adults, but allow to cool before serving. This makes great finger food.

NOTE: Making a quick uncooked tomato passata is as simple as blending fresh seasonal tomatoes together with olive oil, herbs and a little salt and freshly ground black pepper. Store passata in a sealed container in the refrigerator for up to 3 days.

vegetable dishes and sides

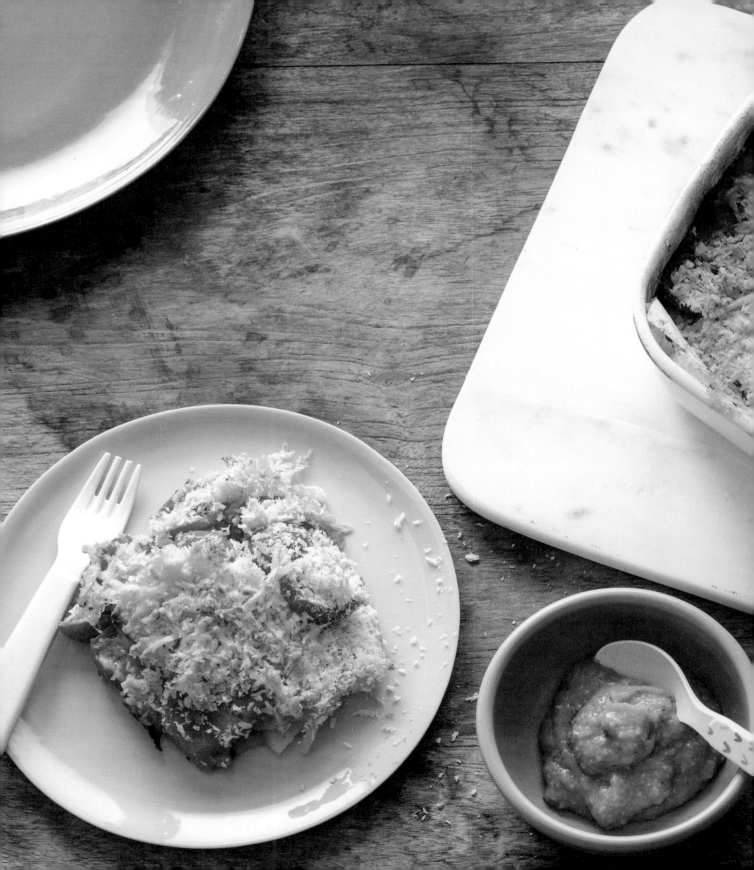

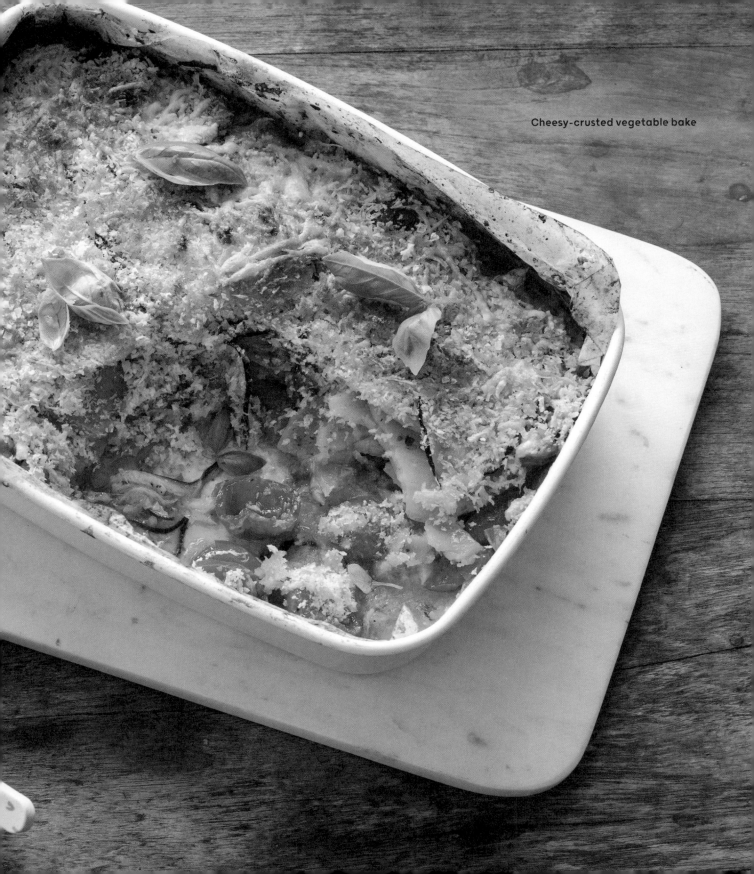

Cheesy-crusted vegetable bake

CHEESY-CRUSTED VEGETABLE BAKE

SERVES 6

PREP TIME: 15 MINUTES

COOKING TIME: 60 MINUTES

A heartwarming dish for the whole family, especially on cooler autumn and winter nights. This is so easy to make and it tastes even better the next day.

400 g (14 oz) pumpkin (squash), peeled and thinly sliced

400 g (14 oz) potatoes, peeled and thinly sliced lengthways

1 zucchini (courgette), sliced diagonally

2 tablespoons melted butter

1 teaspoon mixed dried Italian herbs

sea salt (omit for babies)

freshly ground black pepper (just a tiny amount for babies)

360 g (12½ oz/2 cups) cherry tomatoes (or 400 g/14 oz tinned chopped tomatoes)

50 g (1¾ oz/½ cup) grated parmesan (use ricotta for babies)

60 g (2 oz/½ cup) grated cheddar (use a mild variety for babies)

60 g (2 oz/1 cup) panko (Japanese) breadcrumbs

Preheat the oven to 180°C (350°F). Grease and line a medium baking dish with baking paper.

Place the vegetables in a large mixing bowl. Combine the melted butter and herbs together in another bowl, then toss the mixture through the vegetables, and season with salt and pepper.

Transfer the vegetables to the baking dish in an even layer. Spread the tomatoes over the top. Cover the dish with foil and bake for 45 minutes.

Remove from the oven and take off the foil. Increase the heat of the oven to 200°C (400°F). Top the dish with the cheeses and breadcrumbs, return to the oven and bake for a further 15 minutes, or until the crust is golden and the vegetables are tender when pierced with a knife. Serve hot.

Store in an airtight container in the refrigerator for up to 2 days.

> **For younger babies** thin with a little water and purée until smooth. Allow to cool before serving.
>
> **For older babies** mash to a lumpy texture. Allow to cool before serving.
>
> **For toddlers** serve as for adults, but allow to cool before serving.

DUKKAH SWEET POTATO FRIES WITH YOGHURT-SWEET CHILLI SAUCE

SERVES 4-6

PREP TIME: 5 MINUTES

COOKING TIME: 30 MINUTES

Oven-roasted rather than deep-fried, these fries (chips) are great as a snack or side dish. They are equally delicious made with parsnips or a great waxy potato. Be warned, though, they are addictive. You can also dip the fries in Green goddess avocado dressing (page 204) or Green goddess creamy herb dressing (page 205).

1 kg (2 lb 3 oz) sweet potatoes, peeled, then cut into pieces 1 cm (½ in) wide and 6 cm (2¼ in) long

2 tablespoons macadamia oil (or other cold-pressed oil)

3 teaspoons dukkah (see Note) (omit for babies)

1 teaspoon smoked paprika (just a tiny amount for babies)

¼ teaspoon freshly ground black pepper (just a tiny amount for babies)

1 tablespoon chopped coriander (cilantro) leaves, to serve

1 lime, to serve

YOGHURT-SWEET CHILLI SAUCE

2 tablespoons Greek-style yoghurt

1 teaspoon sweet chilli sauce (omit for babies)

Preheat the oven to 180°C (350°F). Line 2 baking trays with baking paper.

Toss the sweet potatoes in the macadamia oil to coat.

Mix the dukkah, paprika and pepper in a large bowl. Roll the fries in the spice mix and dust off any excess. **(For babies under 12 months leave the spice mixture off the fries.)** Transfer to the lined baking trays and bake until crisp, rotating occasionally, for about 20-30 minutes. Do not let the dukkah burn! Depending on your oven you may want to reduce the heat.

Meanwhile, to make the yoghurt-sweet chilli sauce, mix the ingredients together with a fork in a small bowl. Set aside.

Serve the hot fries with the sauce for dipping, topped with the coriander and a squeeze of lime juice. Store in an airtight container in the refrigerator for up to 2 days.

> **For younger babies** purée the roasted sweet potatoes (without any spice mix) until smooth - thin with a little water if the texture is too thick. Allow to cool before serving.
>
> **For older babies** mash the unspiced fries to a lumpy texture. Allow to cool before serving. Serve with yoghurt without the chilli sauce.
>
> **For toddlers** serve as for adults, but allow to cool before serving.

NOTE: Dukkah is available at most supermarkets. It is usually made up of cumin, coriander, sesame seeds, salt, dried herbs and tree nuts or peanuts.

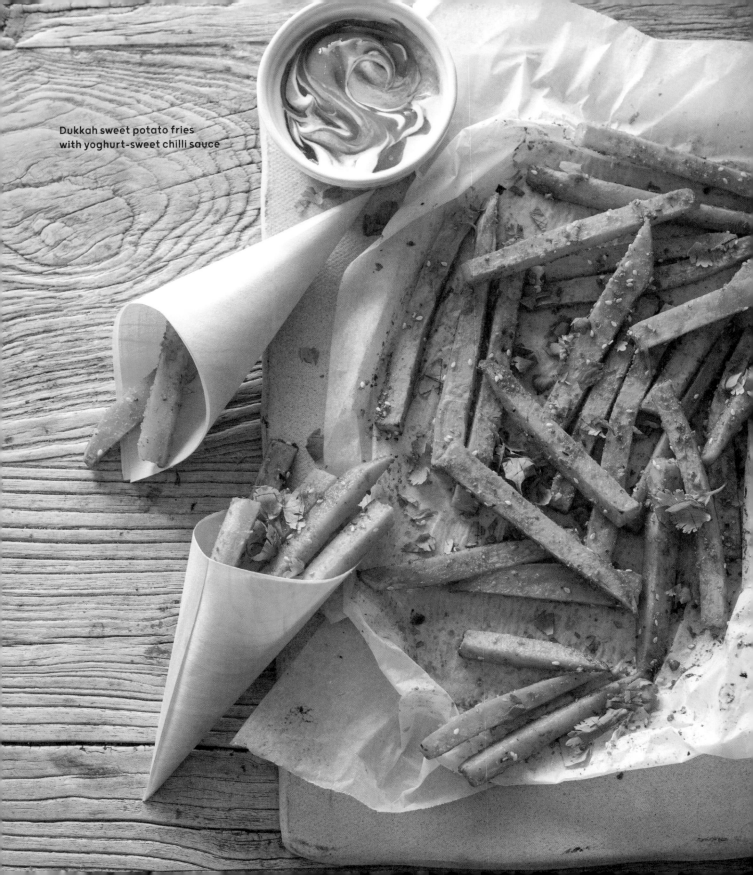

Dukkah sweet potato fries
with yoghurt-sweet chilli sauce

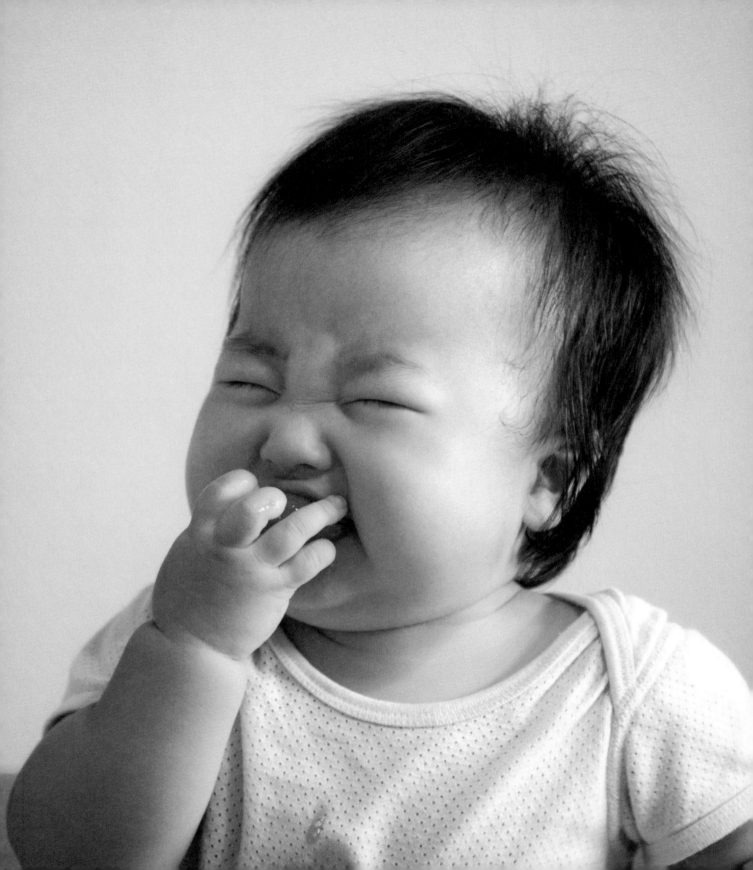

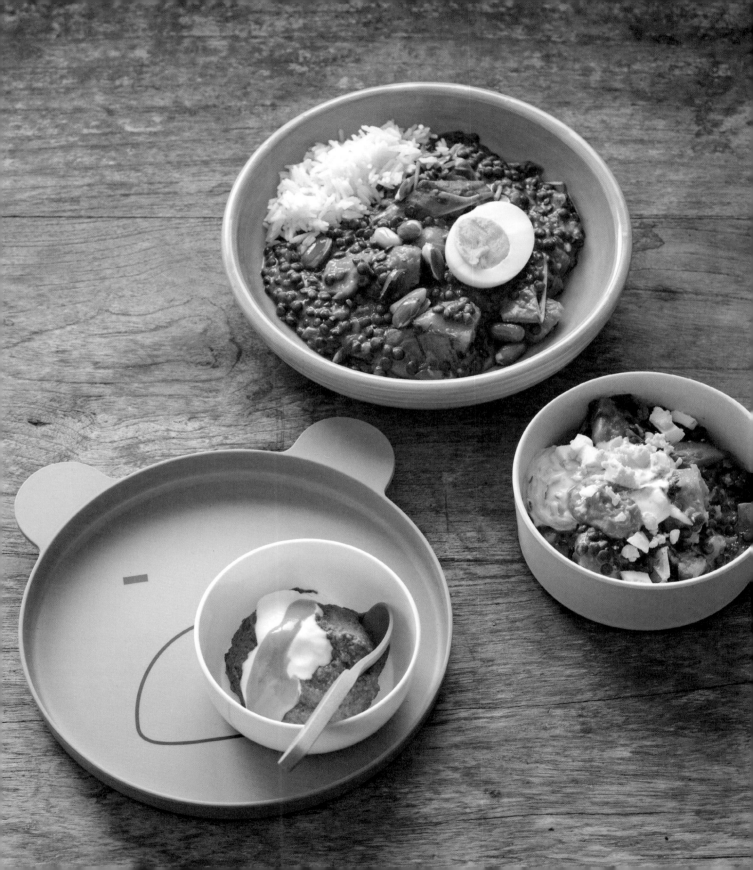

GENTLE INDIAN CURRY OF PUMPKIN AND GREEN LENTILS

SERVES 4

PREP TIME: 10 MINUTES, PLUS OVERNIGHT SOAKING

COOKING TIME: 65 MINUTES

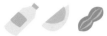

Like most curries, this tastes even better when reheated the next day. Curries freeze well and can be frozen in small amounts, which is handy and economical. Serve the curry with steamed rice and your favourite condiment, such as plain yoghurt with grated cucumber.

80 g (2¾ oz) ghee

2 spring onions (scallions), thinly sliced

2 green chillies, deseeded and finely chopped (omit for babies)

½ teaspoon caraway seeds

¼ teaspoon fenugreek seeds

250 g (9 oz) green lentils, soaked overnight, drained (we like the small Puy lentils)

1 tablespoon tomato paste (concentrated purée)

1 teaspoon mustard seeds

¼ teaspoon ground coriander

250 g (9 oz) pumpkin (squash), skin and seeds removed, roughly chopped into small chunks

500 ml (17 fl oz/2 cups) water or quality vegetable or chicken stock (preferably preservative and additive free)

400 ml (13½ fl oz) coconut cream

sea salt (omit for babies)

100 g (3½ oz/2 cups) baby English spinach leaves

steamed rice, to serve

1 hard-boiled egg, halved, to serve

crushed roasted peanuts (or smooth, unsalted peanut butter for babies – see Home-made nut butters on page 217), to serve

Heat the ghee in a medium heavy-based saucepan over medium-low heat. Add the spring onion and chilli and cook for 2 minutes until slightly soft and translucent. Stir in the caraway and fenugreek seeds and fry for about 2 minutes. Add the lentils, tomato paste, mustard seeds, ground coriander and pumpkin. Add the water or stock and bring to the boil, then reduce the heat, add the coconut cream and simmer for about 1 hour, or until the lentils and pumpkin are tender. Season as required, then gently stir in the spinach leaves.

Serve with steamed rice, and topped with the halved hard-boiled egg and crushed peanuts.

Store in an airtight container in the refrigerator for up to 2 days, or freeze for up to 3 months.

For younger babies purée until smooth with a little steamed rice or pilaf. Add a teaspoon of plain yoghurt and a dollop of smooth, unsalted peanut butter. Allow to cool before serving.

For older babies mash with pilaf or some steamed rice. Serve with plain yoghurt and a dollop of smooth, unsalted peanut butter. Allow to cool before serving.

For toddlers top the curry with chopped hard-boiled egg, yoghurt and finely chopped peanuts or a dollop of peanut butter. Allow to cool before serving.

RED LENTIL DAL

SERVES 6

PREP TIME: 5 MINUTES

COOKING TIME: 40 MINUTES

This is an absolute staple recipe that my husband, Martin, has always cooked in our house. It's better the next day, so make lots! Once you've nailed cooking your dal, you'll find it to be the ultimate nurturing bowl when paired with rice or served as a side dish with a great curry. It's also perfect with yoghurt, Indian breads (roti, naan or poppadoms), chutneys and pickles. This is a delicious gentle-on-the-tummy dal.

20 g (¾ oz) ghee, grapeseed oil or other neutral-flavoured oil
½ large brown onion, thinly sliced
1 garlic clove, finely chopped (just a tiny amount for babies)
1 teaspoon grated fresh ginger
½ teaspoon ground turmeric
250 g (9 oz/1 cup) red lentils, rinsed and drained (see Note)
sea salt (omit for babies)
½ teaspoon garam masala (omit for babies)

Heat the ghee in a medium saucepan over medium heat. Add the onion, garlic and ginger. Reduce the heat a little and cook gently, stirring, for 5–8 minutes until golden brown and soft. Add the turmeric and stir well. Add the drained lentils and fry for several minutes, stirring constantly to prevent sticking. Add 500 ml (17 fl oz/2 cups) water, cover and bring to the boil. Reduce the heat to low and simmer for 15 minutes.

Add a tiny pinch of salt and the garam masala and stir. Cover the pan, reduce the heat to low and cook for another 15–20 minutes, stirring occasionally, until the lentils are soft and the consistency is like porridge - if the dal is too thick, add a little more water; if there's too much liquid, remove the lid and allow the water to cook off. Check the seasoning and add salt as required before serving.

Store in an airtight container in the refrigerator for up to 2 days, or freeze for up to 3 months.

NOTE: Red lentils don't need soaking, but do make sure you rinse them thoroughly before cooking. Discard any lentils that are discoloured or that float to the top of the water.

> **For younger babies** thin the dal with a little water and purée until smooth. Top with a dollop of plain yoghurt. Allow to cool before serving.
>
> **For older babies** serve with a side of plain yoghurt. Allow to cool before serving.
>
> **For toddlers** serve as for adults. If desired, include some yoghurt and a sweet mango chutney with roti bread for dipping. Allow to cool before serving.

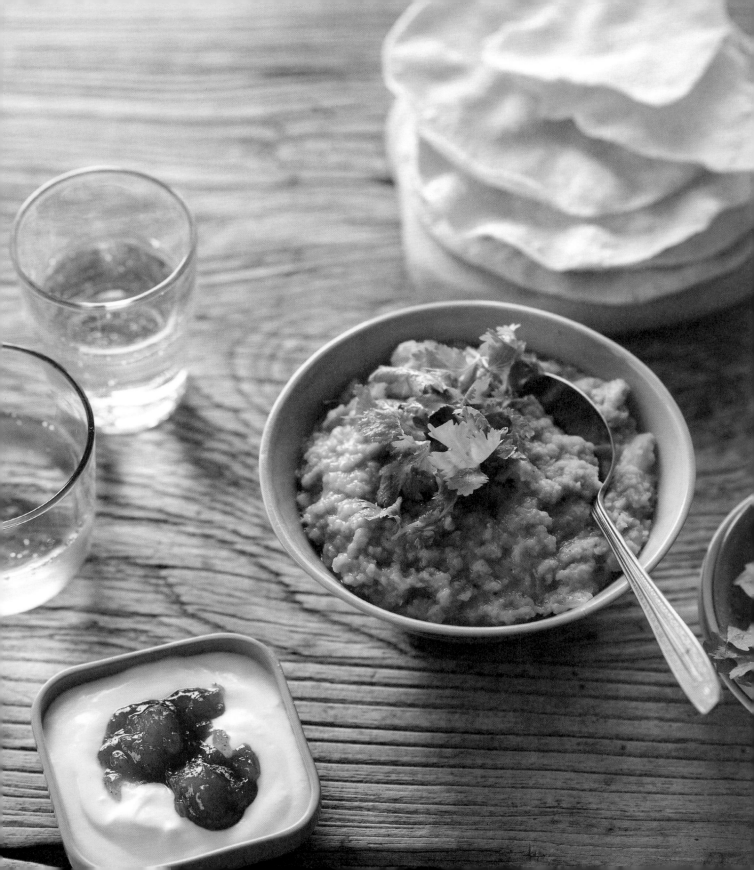

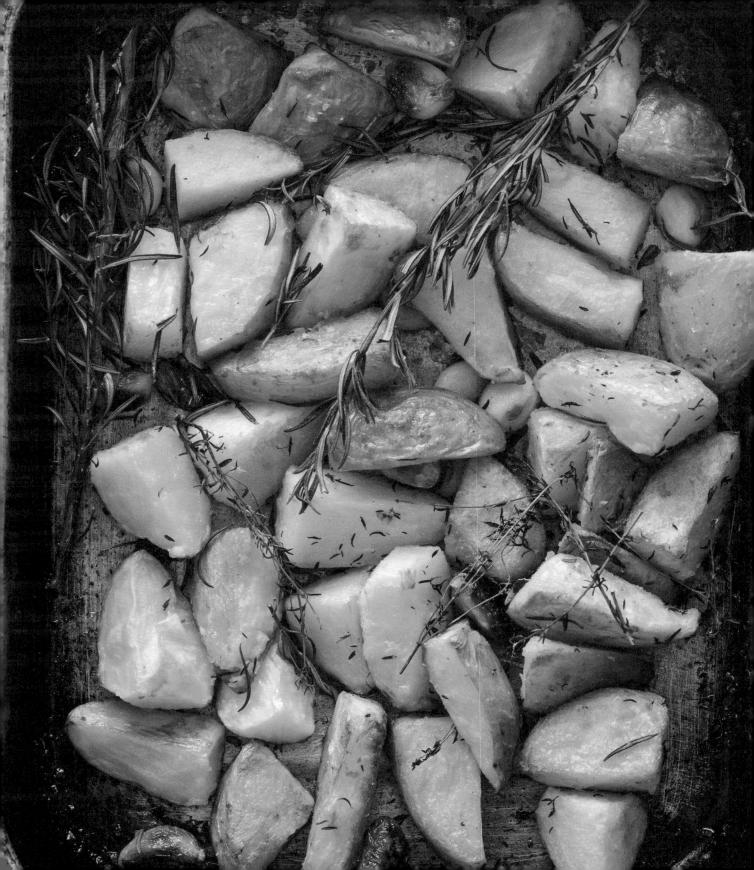

CRISPY ROAST POTATOES WITH GARLIC AND HERBS

SERVES 6-8

PREP TIME: 5 MINUTES

COOKING TIME: 50 MINUTES

Use your favourite roasting potato, but we strongly recommend Dutch creams or kipflers (fingerlings) – something sturdy and waxy is best. For a roasting oil use any quality cold-pressed oil. We prefer macadamia oil, as it gives a smoother buttery flavour. These potatoes make a great addition to Bubble and squeak (page 74).

1 kg (2 lb 3 oz) roasting potatoes, washed and cut into 5 cm (2 in) pieces (no need to peel)
sea salt (omit for babies)
80 ml (2¼ fl oz/⅓ cup) macadamia oil
8 garlic cloves
4 rosemary sprigs
8 thyme sprigs

Put the potatoes in a saucepan of cold salted water and bring to the boil. Once it boils, cook for 5 minutes, then drain well. Return the potatoes to the pan, put the lid on and, holding the lid down firmly, shake the potatoes well for a few seconds so the outsides break up a little and go fluffy. Leave them in the pan to steam-dry.

Meanwhile, preheat the oven to 200°C (400°F). Add the oil to a roasting tin and put it in the oven for a minute to heat. Remove the tin from the oven and add the potatoes, along with the garlic, herbs and a good pinch of salt, and stir to coat. Make sure the potatoes have a little space between them and are not too crowded in the tin, then roast for 20 minutes.

Remove the tin from the oven, turn the potatoes and increase the temperature to 220°C (430°F). Roast for a further 20 minutes, or until the potatoes are brown and crisp, turning once more in the process. Serve sprinkled with a little extra salt. Store in an airtight container in the refrigerator for up to 2 days.

For younger babies remove the garlic and herb sprigs, thin with a little milk and purée the potatoes until smooth. Allow to cool before serving.

For older babies these make perfect finger food provided you remove any hard crunchy pieces, which are a choking hazard. You may need to squash the potato cubes down a bit to make it easier for your baby to chew. Allow to cool before serving.

For toddlers remove any small hard crunchy bits, which are a choking hazard, then serve as for adults, but allow to cool before serving.

WILTED LEAFY GREENS WITH ANCHOVIES

SERVES 4

PREP TIME: 5 MINUTES

COOKING TIME: 5 MINUTES

OPTIONAL

Fast, simple, and utterly delicious and nutritious. The quick wilting of the leafy greens retains their colour, flavour and texture, and most importantly their healthy qualities. Serve this as a side dish with meat and fish. It's also perfect served with polenta, pasta or steamed rice.

2 tablespoons olive oil

4 anchovies, chopped (omit for babies)

2 handfuls of English spinach (baby spinach is fine too)

½ bunch curly kale, roughly chopped

½ Chinese cabbage (wombok), roughly chopped

sea salt (omit for babies)

ground white pepper (just a tiny amount for babies)

Heat the olive oil in a large saucepan over medium heat. Add the anchovies and let them melt down for 1 minute. Add the greens, season lightly with salt and white pepper and stir everything together. Cover the pan with a lid, reduce the heat to low and leave to wilt for 2 minutes.

> **For younger babies** purée the greens (without anchovies) until smooth, and serve with polenta or mashed potato. Allow to cool before serving.
>
> **For older babies** mash the greens (without anchovies) and serve with polenta, mashed potato or steamed rice. Allow to cool before serving.
>
> **For toddlers** serve as for adults, but allow to cool before serving.

MASHED POTATO WITH LEEK AND DILL

SERVES 4-6

PREP TIME: 5 MINUTES

COOKING TIME: 30 MINUTES

An easy, delicious side, and a twist on regular mash, that makes a perfect accompaniment to meat and seafood dishes. It also goes brilliantly in Bubble and squeak (page 74). Puréed, this makes a great first food for babies.

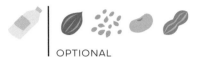

OPTIONAL

2 tablespoons olive oil

1 large leek, white part only, cleaned well and roughly chopped

2 large non-waxy potatoes, peeled and finely diced

500 ml (17 fl oz/2 cups) quality chicken stock (preferably preservative and additive free)

120 g (4¼ oz) thick (double/heavy) cream or full-fat plain yoghurt

1 tablespoon chopped dill

sea salt (omit for babies)

freshly ground black pepper (just a tiny amount for babies)

Tasty toasted sprinkle (page 220), to serve (optional)

Warm the olive oil in a medium saucepan over medium-high heat. Add the leek and sauté until soft, about 5 minutes. Add the potatoes, stock and 500 ml (17 fl oz/2 cups) water and bring to the boil. Reduce the heat to low and simmer until the potatoes are very soft, about 20 minutes.

Remove the pan from the heat and drain the potatoes, reserving the stock. Add the cream or yoghurt and dill and mash until slightly lumpy. Add a little stock if the mixture is too dry. Season with salt and pepper to taste. Top with the tasty toasted sprinkle (if using) and serve.

Store in an airtight container in the refrigerator for up to 2 days.

> **For younger babies** purée everything, including the sprinkle, until smooth, and top with puréed wilted greens. Allow to cool before serving.
>
> **For older babies** serve as is, topped with wilted greens. Allow to cool before serving.
>
> **For toddlers** serve as for adults, but allow to cool before serving.

ROAST CINNAMON PUMPKIN

SERVES 4

PREP TIME: 5 MINUTES

COOKING TIME: 35 MINUTES

OPTIONAL

Pumpkin (squash) is one of our favourite vegetables to cook. This recipe is elegantly simple with delicious roasted, nutty flavours. It's great just as is, or you can top it with a sprinkle of crumbled feta cheese. This is a great ingredient for Bubble and squeak (page 74). Puréed, this also makes a great first food for babies.

¼ butternut pumpkin (squash), peeled and deseeded, cut into about 8 wedges
1 teaspoon ground cinnamon (just a tiny amount for babies)
2 tablespoons pepitas (pumpkin seeds)
2 teaspoons sesame seeds
dash of walnut oil or other nut oil, to serve
pinch of salt (omit for babies)

Preheat the oven to 180°C (350°F). Line a baking tray with baking paper.

Toss the pumpkin wedges, cinnamon and pepitas together in a large bowl, then transfer to the baking tray. Roast in the oven for 25-35 minutes or until the pumpkin is tender when pierced with a knife.

Toast the sesame seeds in a dry frying pan over medium heat for about 1 minute until lightly brown - be careful not to burn them.

Sprinkle the pumpkin with the toasted sesame seeds. Serve warm with a drizzle of nut oil and season with a little salt if required.

Store in an airtight container in the refrigerator for up to 2 days.

For younger babies purée until smooth, with some ricotta if desired, and allow to cool before serving.

For older babies mash coarsely or cut into finger food-sized pieces. Allow to cool before serving.

For toddlers serve as for adults, but allow to cool before serving.

SWEET POTATO MASH WITH GINGER AND COCONUT

SERVES 4

PREP TIME: 5 MINUTES

COOKING TIME: 25 MINUTES

OPTIONAL

There is so much flavour in this recipe. Sweet potato is a much undervalued vegetable, and once you try this mash it's sure to become a favourite.

1 tablespoon cold-pressed sunflower oil or use a nut oil
20 g (¾ oz) butter or ghee
½ small brown onion, finely chopped
1 teaspoon finely chopped fresh ginger
2 sweet potatoes, peeled and chopped into 2 cm (¾ in) cubes
400 ml (13½ fl oz) quality vegetable stock (preferably preservative and additive free)
400 ml (13½ fl oz) coconut cream
sea salt (omit for babies)
1 tablespoon finely chopped coriander (cilantro)

Warm the oil and butter together in a medium saucepan over medium-high heat. Add the onion and ginger and sauté until soft, about 5 minutes. Add the sweet potato and stock and bring to the boil. Reduce the heat to low and simmer until the sweet potato is soft, about 20 minutes.

Remove from the heat, pour off the liquid and allow to cool before mashing with the coconut cream. Season with salt if required.

To serve, reheat gently and garnish with the coriander.

Store in an airtight container in the refrigerator for up to 2 days.

> **For younger babies** purée until smooth and allow to cool before serving.
>
> **For older babies** serve as is with a drizzle of coconut cream. Allow to cool before serving.
>
> **For toddlers** serve as for adults, but allow to cool before serving.

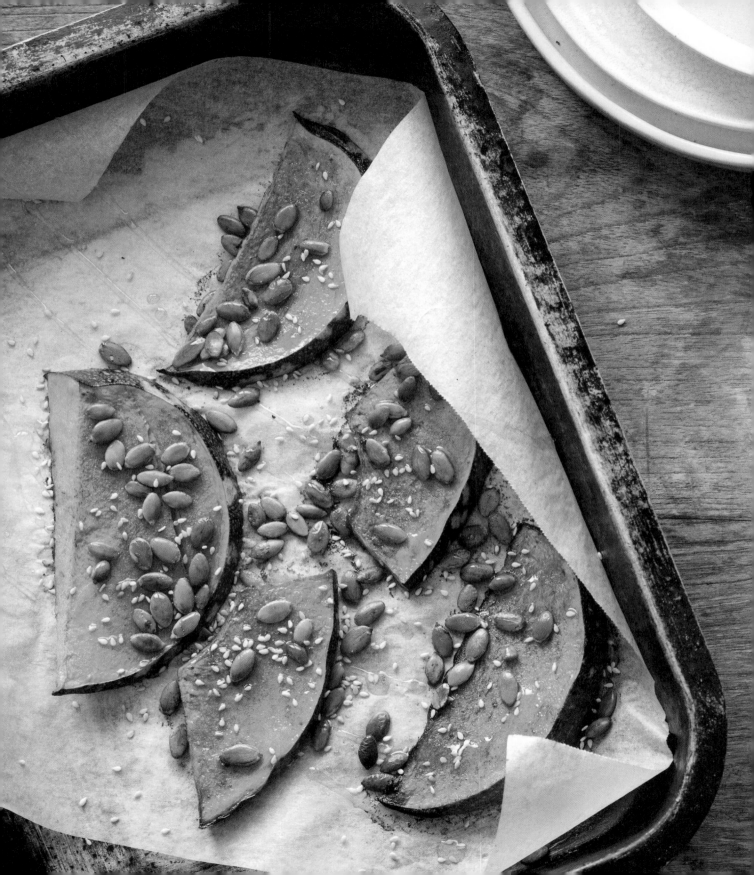

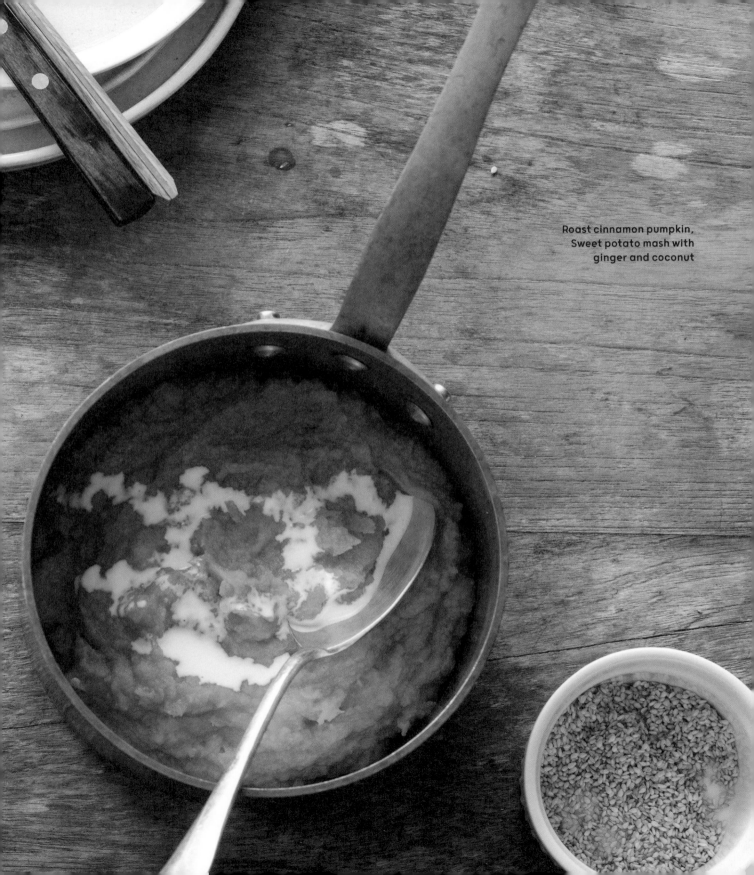

Roast cinnamon pumpkin,
Sweet potato mash with
ginger and coconut

CANNELLINI BEANS WITH ROASTED GARLIC, MISO AND PARSLEY

SERVES 4-6

PREP TIME: 5 MINUTES

COOKING TIME: 15 MINUTES

OPTIONAL

A perfect side with grilled fish or poultry, this also makes a nourishing breakfast spread on toast – for extra deliciousness top with a poached egg. Puréed, this is a great protein-rich food for young babies.

1 tablespoon olive oil

½ small brown onion, finely chopped

800 g (1 lb 12 oz) tinned cannellini beans, rinsed and drained

2 roasted garlic cloves (you can use less for babies) (see Note)

1 teaspoon white miso (omit for babies)

2 tablespoons finely chopped flat-leaf (Italian) parsley

sea salt (omit for babies)

freshly ground black pepper (just a tiny amount for babies)

Heat the olive oil in a small saucepan over medium-low heat. Add the onion and sauté until translucent, 5-7 minutes. Now add the cannellini beans and roasted garlic. (Set aside baby's portion now.)

Mix the miso with 50 ml (1¾ fl oz) water to make a paste, add it to the beans, then mash lightly. Fold in the parsley. Add salt and pepper to taste - but you may find there is ample seasoning from the miso. Serve warm.

Store in an airtight container in the refrigerator for up to 2 days, or freeze for up to 3 months.

> **For younger babies** purée until smooth. Allow to cool before serving.
>
> **For older babies** serve as is with a drizzle of coconut cream. Allow to cool before serving.
>
> **For toddlers** serve as for adults, but allow to cool before serving.

NOTE: For roasted garlic, preheat the oven to 170°C (340°F). Toss a whole garlic bulb in ½ tablespoon olive oil, place it on a baking tray lined with baking paper, then roast for about 20 minutes or until soft. When cool, peel and set aside. Roasting garlic ahead of time is a great idea, as it's an easy, delicious and healthy go-to item in your refrigerator. It will enhance any vegetable purée and is much gentler in flavour than raw garlic.

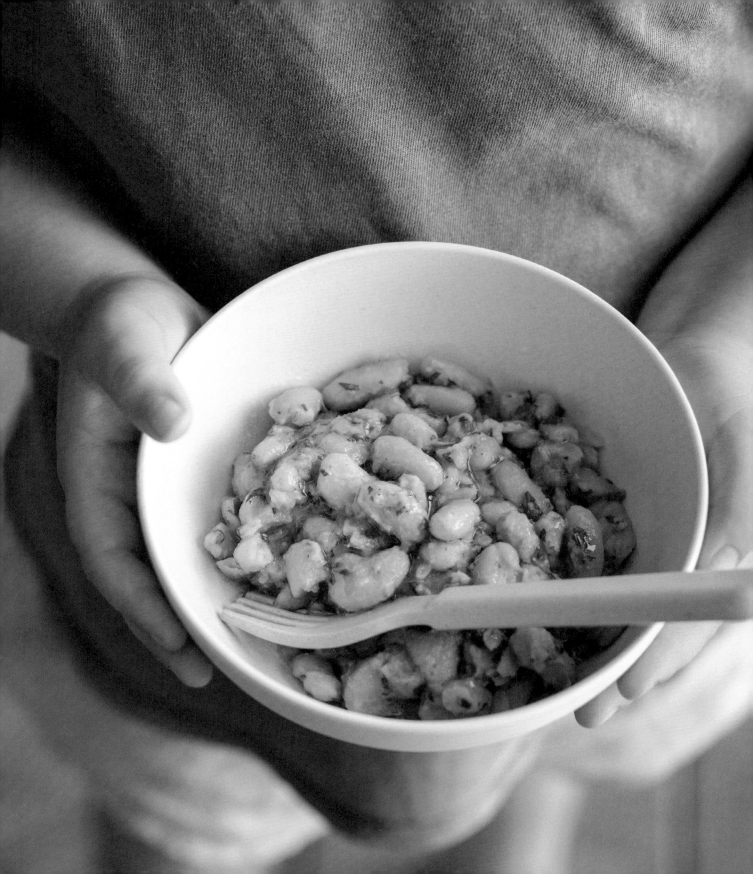

meat
and fish

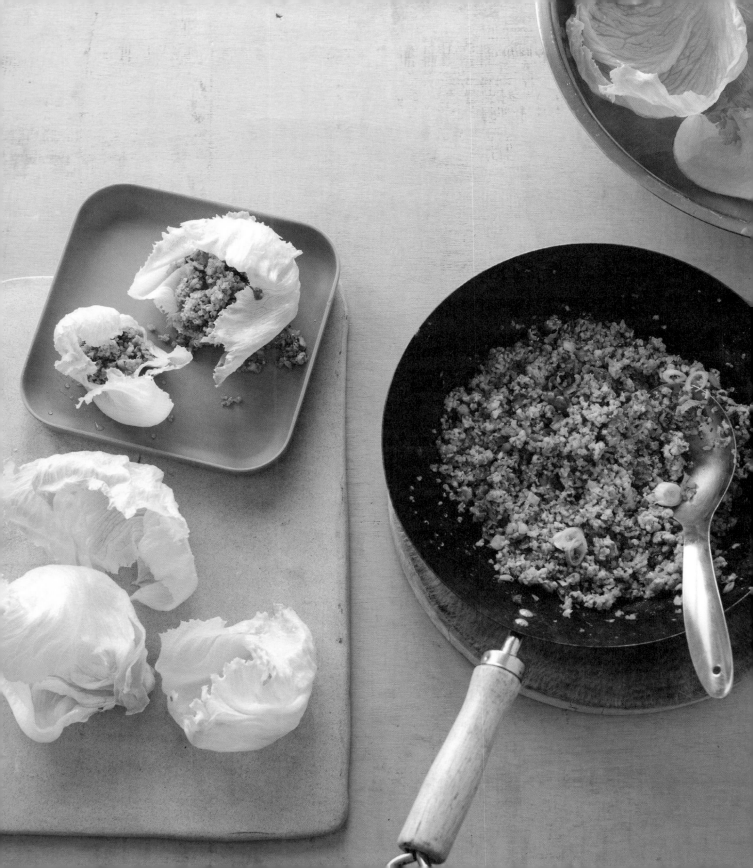

SAN CHOI BAO WITH QUINOA, PEANUTS AND CHICKEN

OPTIONAL

Healthy and full of flavour, this protein-rich variation on a Chinese classic will please everyone. The dish lends itself to so many great ingredients. Swap out the chicken for prawns (shrimp), minced (ground) pork or diced tofu, or add some shredded omelette, and mix up the herbs.

200 g (7 oz/1 cup) white quinoa, well rinsed and drained
1 tablespoon peanut oil or cold-pressed sunflower oil
1 garlic clove, crushed (just a tiny amount for babies)
1 tablespoon minced fresh ginger
40 g (1¼ oz/¼ cup) peanuts, finely chopped
4 spring onions (scallions), thinly sliced
250 g (9 oz) minced (ground) chicken (or mince/grind 2 skinless boneless chicken thighs in a food processor)
½ teaspoon ground cumin
¼ teaspoon ground coriander
1 tablespoon soy sauce (omit for babies)
dash of shaoxing rice wine, or use sherry vinegar or red-wine vinegar or a quality chicken stock (preferably preservative and additive free)
2 tablespoons roughly chopped coriander (cilantro) leaves
1 tablespoon store-bought Asian fried shallots (optional)
6 iceberg lettuce leaf cups, washed and dried (from 1 iceberg lettuce)
Almond, ginger and coconut sauce (page 210), to serve (omit for babies)
Peanut sauce (for adults) or Peanut sauce for baby (page 211), to serve

Place the quinoa in a medium saucepan. Cover with 250 ml (8½ fl oz/1 cup) water, set over medium-high heat and bring to the boil. Immediately reduce the heat and simmer until all the water has been absorbed and the quinoa seeds have started to become translucent. Remove from the heat and cover the pan with a clean tea towel (dish towel) folded in half underneath the lid (see Note). Set aside (reserve a few teaspoons of cooked quinoa for baby).

Heat the oil in a wok over high heat. Add the garlic, ginger, peanuts and half the spring onion and toss well until fragrant and starting to colour. Remove from the wok and set aside.

Add the chicken to the wok and stir-fry until well cooked and lightly browned. (Set some chicken mixture aside for baby now.)

Add the cumin, coriander, soy sauce and rice wine, then toss to coat the chicken and stir-fry for a further 30 seconds - make sure you cook off the alcohol from the rice wine if serving to babies, or just use stock. Add the peanut mixture and heat through for about 30 seconds.

Remove from the heat and fold through the coriander and quinoa to warm them through.

Spoon the san choi bao mixture onto a platter and sprinkle with the remaining spring onion and the fried shallots, if using. Spoon the mixture into lettuce cups before eating with the sauces.

Store the cooked mixture in an airtight container in the refrigerator for up to 2 days - but serve on fresh lettuce leaves.

>

For younger babies thin some of the chicken mixture with a little water and reserved quinoa, and purée until smooth. Allow to cool before serving.

For older babies this makes great finger food. Allow to cool before serving.

For toddlers serve as for adults. Allow to cool before serving.

NOTE: This tea towel trick allows the excess steam and moisture to be absorbed and keeps the quinoa warm so you will have fluffy quinoa every time. Try this bulletproof technique for rice cooked with the absorption method too.

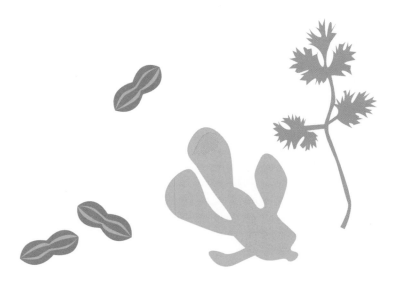

RICE PAPER ROLLS WITH PRAWNS, MINT AND OMELETTE

These popular rolls are super healthy and, once you've got the knack of rice-paper rolling, you'll discover they can hold many different fillings. Feel free to use shredded chicken, pork or beef instead of prawns, or make it vegan with thinly sliced cucumber, tofu and avocado. The hardest thing here is the wrapping and rolling – it can make for hilarious family fun, but don't add too much filling, and remember patience is everything!

OPTIONAL

1 teaspoon butter or sunflower oil
2 eggs, beaten
125 ml (4 fl oz/½ cup) warm water
8 large rice paper sheets
8 cooked king prawns (jumbo shrimp), peeled and deveined, sliced in half or cut into thin slices
140 g (5 oz/1 cup) rice vermicelli noodles, soaked in boiling water until al dente, drained
2 handfuls of shredded iceberg lettuce
1 carrot, grated
1 tablespoon chopped Vietnamese mint
Peanut sauce (for adults) or Peanut sauce for baby (page 211), to serve
Coconut lime dressing (page 214) (omit for babies)

Heat the butter or oil in a frying pan over low heat. Add the beaten egg and spread it over the pan in a thin layer. Cook very gently, just heating the egg through until opaque and cooked. Remove from the heat and set aside to cool. Cut the egg into thin slices.

Add the warm water to a wide shallow bowl. Dip a rice paper wrapper into the water for about 5 seconds, until just translucent but not too soft. Transfer it to a plate where it will soften further.

To assemble a roll, put 2 prawn halves on the lower third of the rice paper, leaving about 2 cm (¾ in) gap at the bottom of the wrapper. Top with small amounts of the rice vermicelli, omelette, lettuce, carrot and mint in a neat pile - be careful because if there's too much filling your rice paper roll will self-destruct on rolling!

Fold the bottom of the wrapper over the filling, then hold it in place with one finger and fold both sides in. Gently but snugly, keep rolling up the rest of the wrapper, then press the seam closed. (You might want to wet your fingers when rolling the wrappers, so they don't stick.) Repeat this process with the remaining wrappers and filling.

Cover with a damp cloth to keep them moist.

>

Serve with peanut sauce and coconut lime dressing, or your favourite dipping sauce.

Store the prepared rice paper rolls in an airtight container in the refrigerator for up to 24 hours. Ideally leave space between rolls and layer them between sheets of baking paper to prevent them sticking together.

For older babies this is perfect finger food. Make sure the ingredients are finely chopped to avoid any choking hazard.

For toddlers serve as for adults, but go easy on the spicy sauces until they are ready for stronger flavours.

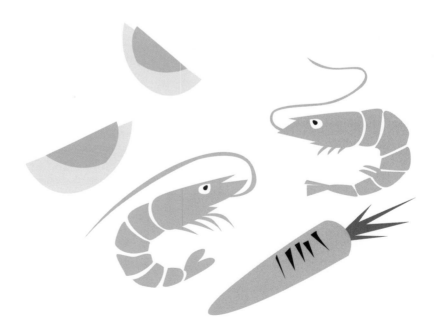

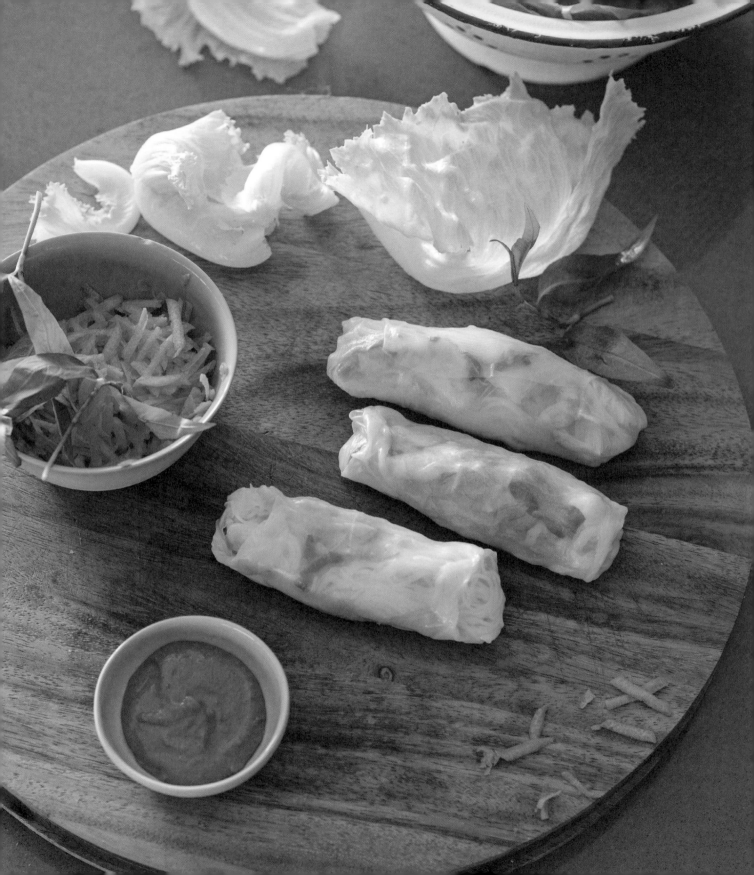

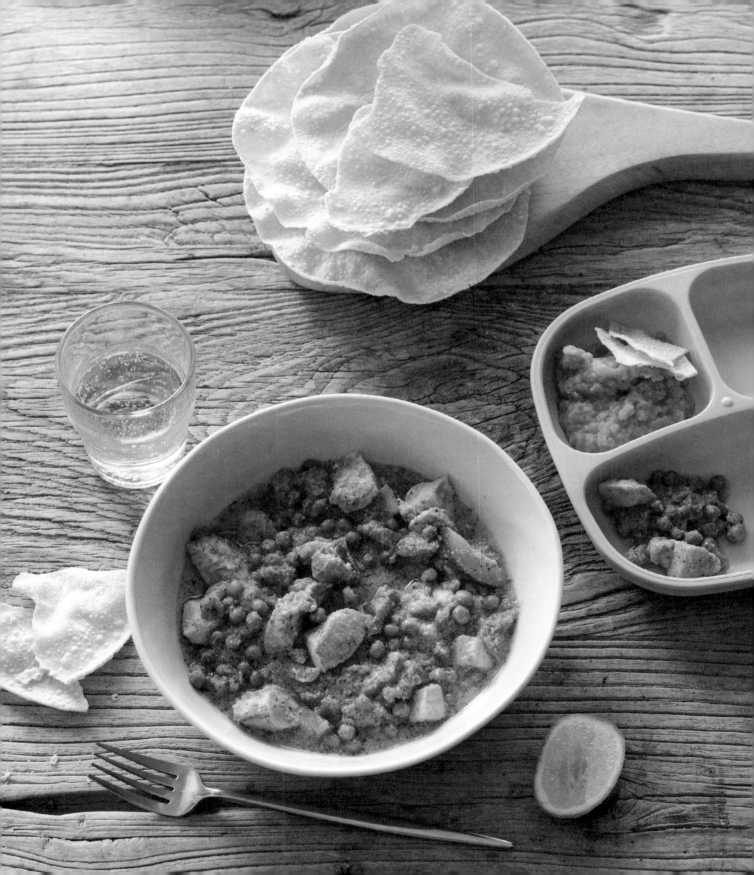

CHICKEN CURRY WITH YOGHURT AND MINT

SERVES 5-6

PREP TIME: 10 MINUTES

COOKING TIME: 35 MINUTES

OPTIONAL

Here's another gentle curry that's so easy to prepare. There are no hot spices so it's perfect for baby and toddler. If you want to spice it up if serving just for adults, add a chilli to the spice paste at the beginning. Serve with poppadoms and a side dish of Red lentil dal (page 132).

10 g (¼ oz/½ cup) mint leaves, plus extra coarsely chopped mint to serve

1 red onion, coarsely chopped

2 garlic cloves (just a tiny amount for babies)

1 teaspoon coarsely chopped fresh ginger

2 tablespoons ghee or macadamia oil

1 teaspoon ground turmeric

1 teaspoon garam masala (just a tiny amount for babies)

125 g (4½ oz/½ cup) plain yoghurt

2 small zucchini (courgettes), coarsely chopped

2 tomatoes, coarsely chopped

1 kg (2 lb 3 oz) skinless boneless chicken thighs, cut into bite-sized pieces

155 g (5½ oz/1 cup) frozen peas, defrosted

salt (omit for babies)

coriander (cilantro) leaves, coarsely chopped, to serve

steamed rice, to serve

lime cheeks, to serve

To make the spice paste, blend the mint, onion, garlic and ginger to a smooth paste in a blender or food processor. Add a little oil if it's too dry.

Heat a large heavy-based saucepan over medium heat and add the ghee. When the ghee is hot add the spice paste. Cook for 5 minutes, stirring gently, until soft and fragrant. Add the turmeric and garam masala and cook for another 2 minutes. Add the yoghurt, zucchini and tomatoes and cook for a further 3 minutes until the liquid starts to reduce. Add the chicken and stir it through to coat it in the mixture. Cover and cook on low heat for 20 minutes, until the chicken is cooked through. Add the peas for the final 5 minutes - you may want to leave the lid off at this stage to reduce the liquid, but leave enough so the curry has its own delicious sauce. (Set aside baby's portion now.)

Season the dish with salt to taste. Top with the chopped mint and coriander and serve with the steamed rice and lime cheeks. Store in an airtight container in the refrigerator for up to 2 days, or freeze for up to 3 months.

For younger babies purée with rice until smooth. Serve with a swirl of yoghurt, if desired. Allow to cool before serving.

For older babies this makes great finger food. Make sure the ingredients are finely chopped to avoid choking hazards. Crumble poppadoms (if using), as these can be sharp. Allow to cool before serving.

For toddlers serve as for adults, but allow to cool before serving.

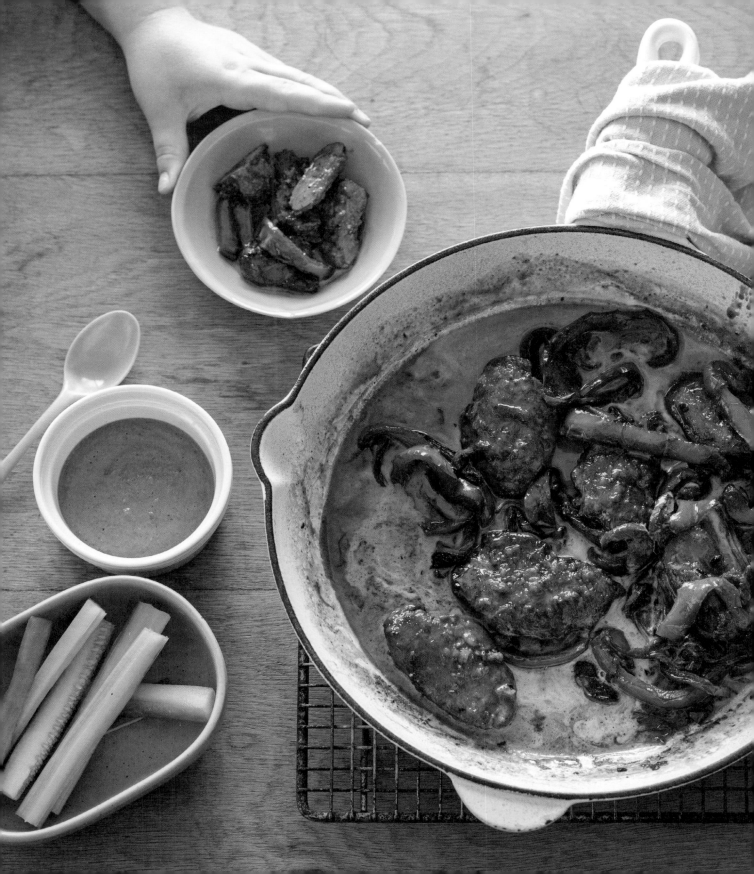

CREAMY CHICKEN LIVERS WITH BRAISED CAPSICUM

SERVES 4

PREP TIME: 5 MINUTES

COOKING TIME: 15 MINUTES

This is arguably one of the most delicious recipes in this book. Serve with gnocchi, polenta or Mashed potato with leek and dill (page 137). The dish is high in vitamin A, so keep portions small for children under 12 months and don't serve it more than once a week.

500 g (1 lb 2 oz) fresh chicken livers, trimmed, rinsed and patted dry
sea salt (omit for babies)
freshly ground black pepper (just a tiny amount for babies)
75 g (2¾ oz/⅓ cup) plain (all-purpose) flour (substitute gluten-free flour if family members are gluten-intolerant or coeliac)
2 tablespoons olive oil
20 g (¾ oz) butter
½ small red onion, thinly sliced
1 large green capsicum (bell pepper), halved, deseeded and very thinly sliced
3 tablespoons sherry vinegar
125 ml (4 fl oz/½ cup) Marsala
125 ml (4 fl oz/½ cup) quality chicken stock (preferably preservative and additive free) or water
3 tablespoons pouring (single/light) cream

Season the chicken livers lightly with salt and pepper, then dust liberally with the flour. Shake off the excess.

Add half the olive oil and half the butter to a large frying pan set over medium heat. When the butter is bubbling, increase the heat to high, add half the livers and fry for 2 minutes on each side, so they are nicely coloured but still pink on the inside. Transfer the livers to a plate, cover with foil and set aside while you cook the remaining livers in the remaining butter.

While all the cooked livers are resting, return the pan to medium heat. Add the remaining olive oil along with the onion, capsicum and a pinch of salt. Cook, stirring, for about 6 minutes until the vegetables are soft, golden and well caramelised. Add the sherry vinegar, Marsala, and stock or water and stir through. Turn the heat down a little and simmer until the liquid is reduced by half. The wine will cook off and bring out the natural sugars in the dish. Add the cream and return the livers to the pan. Check the seasoning and stir gently over high heat for 30 seconds until heated through. Store in an airtight container in the refrigerator for up to 24 hours.

For younger babies purée until smooth - add a little water to dilute if it's too thick. Allow to cool before serving.

For older babies blitz until coarse or, if your baby is ready for finger food, cut it into small bite-sized pieces for little hands to grab. Allow to cool before serving.

For toddlers chop into bite-sized pieces and add a few carrot, cucumber or celery sticks to use as dippers for the sauce. Allow to cool before serving.

MEATLOAF WITH MAPLE-MISO GLAZE

OPTIONAL

Using quality minced (ground) beef with a good fat ratio will help to hold the meatloaf together. For a firmer loaf, use an extra egg. Serve with Mashed potato with leek and dill (page 137). The glaze also makes a great barbecue sauce.

80 g (2¾ oz/1 cup) fresh or 100 g (3½ oz/ 1 cup) dried breadcrumbs (or 100 g/ 3½ oz/1 cup ground almonds to make it gluten-free)

90 g (3 oz/⅓ cup) sour cream

1 tablespoon olive oil

1 large brown onion, finely chopped

2 garlic cloves, finely chopped

3 tablespoons worcestershire sauce (omit for babies)

1 teaspoon dijon mustard

3 tablespoons tomato paste (concentrated purée)

2 tablespoons finely chopped flat-leaf (Italian) parsley

freshly ground black pepper (just a tiny amount for babies)

2 large eggs, beaten

2 kg (4 lb 6 oz) minced (ground) beef

GLAZE (OMIT FOR BABIES)

2 tablespoons tomato paste (concentrated purée)

2 tablespoons worcestershire sauce

2 dessertspoons maple syrup

1½ teaspoons miso

juice of 1 lemon

Combine the breadcrumbs and sour cream in a bowl and allow to stand for 15 minutes. Preheat the oven to 180°C (350°F). Grease and line a loaf (bar) tin with baking paper.

Heat the olive oil in a large frying pan, add the onion and garlic and cook gently until translucent and soft, about 6-7 minutes. Remove from the heat, transfer to a small bowl and allow to cool. Add the onion mixture to the breadcrumb mixture.

In a large mixing bowl, combine the worcestershire sauce, mustard and tomato paste, then add the parsley and season well with black pepper. Add the breadcrumb mixture, along with the beaten egg and the beef and mix well. Transfer to the tin and bake in the oven for 30 minutes.

To make the glaze, whisk all the ingredients together.

Remove the meatloaf from the oven and spread the glaze over the top using the back of a spoon. Bake in the oven for another 30 minutes. Test the meatloaf with a skewer - the juices should run clear and the loaf should feel firm. Remove from the oven and allow to rest for 10 minutes before slicing, giving it time to set so it won't crumble when sliced. Store in an airtight container in the refrigerator for up to 2 days, or freeze for up to 3 months.

For younger babies purée the meatloaf (not using the glazed area) with some mashed potato until smooth - add milk to dilute if it's too thick. Allow to cool before serving.

For older babies this makes ideal finger food - just crumble it up. You can also mix it through mashed potato or vegetable purée. Allow to cool before serving.

For toddlers serve as for adults, but allow to cool before serving.

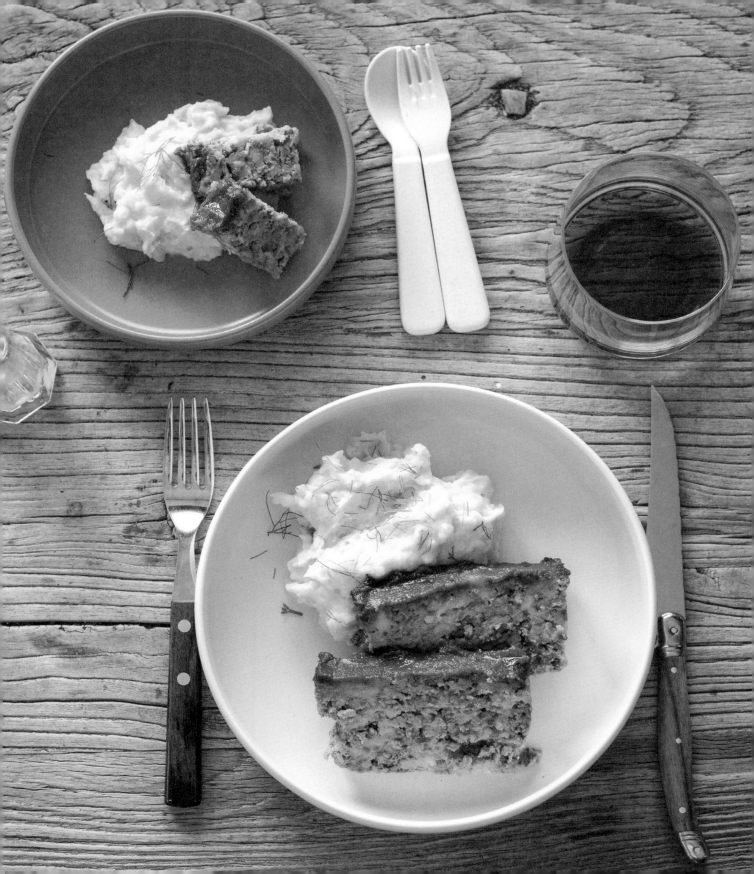

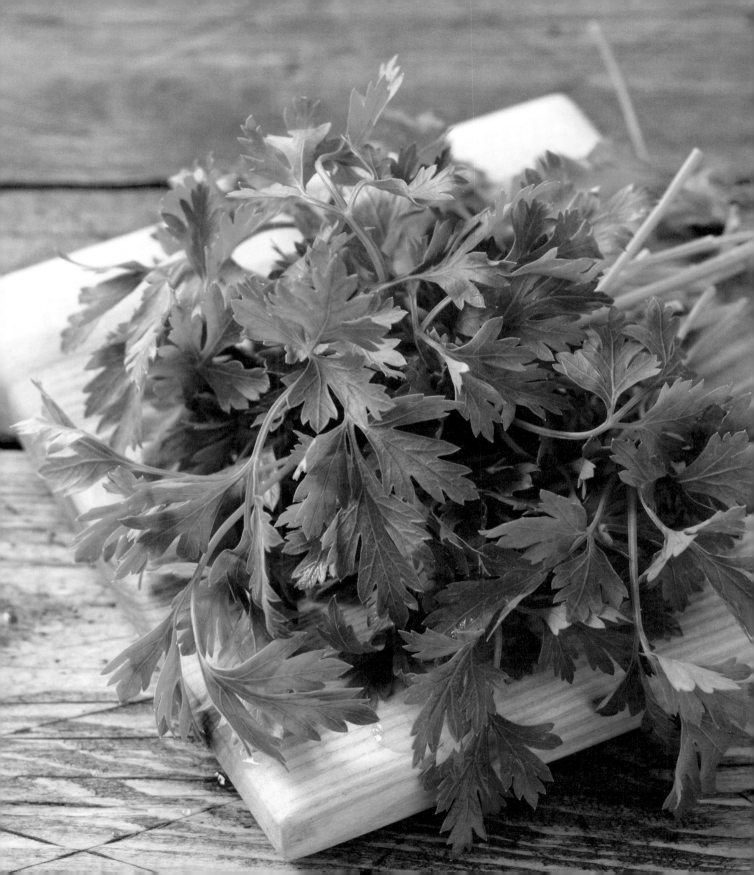

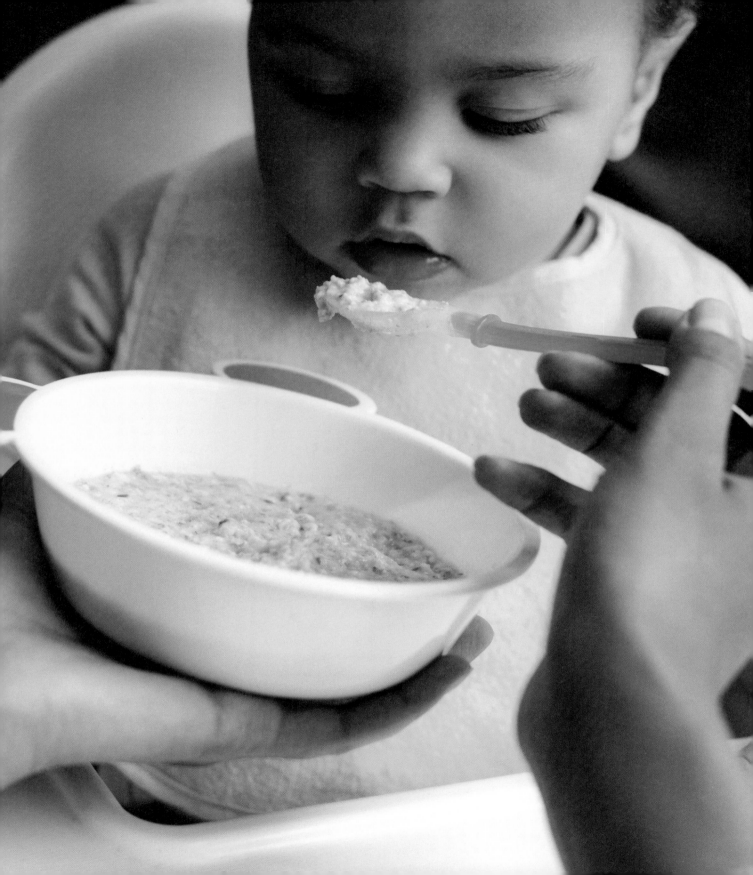

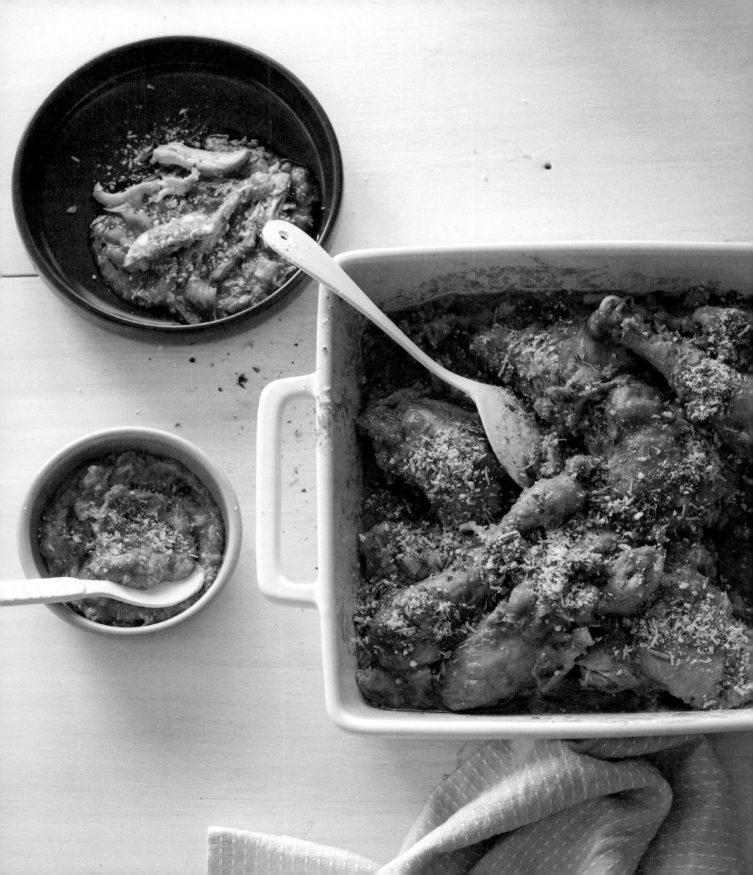

SIMPLE CHICKEN CASSEROLE WITH CHEESY NUT CRUMB

The easiest of healthy recipes and a foundation that you can build on again and again, changing the flavour profile as you go. Once you have this down pat, you are bound to make it regularly. You can also use skinless boneless chicken thighs and slow-cook them until the meat falls apart. This casserole freezes well and makes for the perfect emergency 'I forgot to cook' dinner. Use a gluten-free flour if you need to, but do not skip seasoning the flour – it makes such a difference. We love serving this with mashed potatoes and steamed greens.

75 g (2¾ oz/½ cup) plain (all-purpose) flour (substitute gluten-free flour if family members are gluten-intolerant or coeliac)
sea salt (omit for babies)
freshly ground black pepper (just a tiny amount for babies)
1 kg (2 lb 3 oz) chicken drumsticks and thighs on the bone
2½ tablespoons olive oil
1 small brown onion, finely diced
2 garlic cloves, crushed
1 carrot, finely diced
2 celery stalks, sliced 1 cm (½ in) thick
1 rosemary sprig, leaves picked
4 thyme sprigs
2 bay leaves
1½ tablespoons tomato paste (concentrated purée)
750 ml (25½ fl oz/3 cups) quality chicken stock (preferably preservative and additive free)
chopped flat-leaf (Italian) parsley, to serve

CHEESY NUT CRUMB
50 g (1¾ oz/½ cup) finely grated parmesan (use ricotta for babies)
40 g (1½ oz/¼ cup) roughly chopped almonds
30 g (1 oz/½ cup) fresh breadcrumbs
1 tablespoon roughly chopped flat-leaf (Italian) parsley,

Place the flour in a large bowl and season well with salt and pepper. Toss the chicken pieces in the flour mixture to coat, then shake off any excess. Set the chicken aside and discard the used flour mixture.

Heat a large heavy-based frying pan over medium heat. Add 2 tablespoons of the olive oil and brown the chicken all over. Remove the chicken from the pan and set aside. Add the remaining oil to the pan along with the onion, garlic, carrot, celery, rosemary, thyme and bay leaves, and sauté over medium-low heat until soft but not brown, about 4 minutes. Stir in the tomato paste, then pour in the stock. Bring to the boil, then reduce the heat to a simmer.

Return the chicken to the pan, cover with a lid and cook for 1 hour or until the chicken is cooked through and starts to fall off the bone.

>

Meanwhile, to make the cheesy nut crumb, preheat the oven to 180°C (350°F) and line a baking tray with baking paper.

Combine all the crumb ingredients in a medium bowl, then transfer to the prepared baking tray. Bake in the oven for 10 minutes, stirring twice during baking to ensure an even golden brown colour.

When the chicken is cooked, discard the bay leaves and thyme stalk, add the parsley and adjust the seasoning as required. Serve sprinkled with the cheesy nut crumb.

Store in an airtight container in the refrigerator for up to 2 days, or freeze for up to 3 months.

For younger babies purée some of the shredded chicken meat with the casserole juices and vegies until smooth. Allow to cool before serving.

For older babies serve the shredded meat as finger food and mash or chop the vegies into tiny pieces. Allow to cool before serving.

For toddlers serve as for adults, but allow to cool before serving. Older toddlers love chicken drumsticks, but watch them while they're eating and keep an eye out for the bones, which can be a choking hazard.

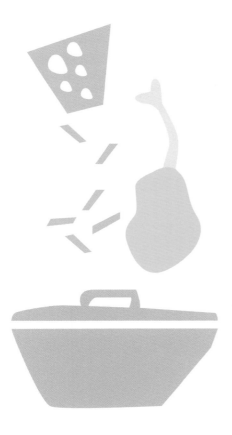

PORK COOKED IN MILK WITH SAGE AND LEMON

SERVES 8-10

PREP TIME: 10 MINUTES

COOKING TIME: 2 HOURS

OPTIONAL

This is so delicious that eating the leftovers the next day is never a bad idea. You really want the pork to sit snugly in the casserole dish or pan so you keep all the moisture in the meat. We like to serve this with blanched greens, such as English spinach, cavolo nero or zucchini (courgette) ribbons, and a big chunk of fresh bread.

olive oil

2 kg (4 lb 6 oz) boneless pork shoulder or neck, skin and excess fat removed, cut into pieces about 5–6 cm (2–2¼ in) thick

sea salt (omit for babies)

10 garlic cloves, peeled

1 large bunch sage leaves (you'll need approximately 1½–2 cups loosely packed leaves)

zest and juice of 2 lemons

1 litre (34 fl oz/4 cups) full-cream (whole) milk

freshly ground black pepper (just a tiny amount for babies)

Preheat the oven to 160°C (320°F).

Place a deep, heavy-based, ovenproof frying pan or flameproof casserole dish over high heat and add a good splash of olive oil. Season the pork with salt, then add the pieces to the pan and brown it well on all sides. When nicely coloured, remove the pork from the pan and set aside.

Reduce the heat slightly and add a splash more oil, followed by the garlic. Toss the garlic well to colour and soften, for about 2 minutes, then add three-quarters of the sage and all the lemon zest. Stir well.

Return the pork to the pan along with the milk, half the lemon juice and a good grinding of pepper. You want your pork to be sitting snugly in the pan and the milk to come about halfway up the pork. Cover the pork with a damp piece of baking paper, then cover the pan with a lid or fitted piece of foil. Place the pork into the oven to slowly braise. Cook for about 2 hours until tender, checking and turning after 1 hour. When the pork is cooked it will be soft and falling apart and the milky sauce will be golden and deliciously curdled. Remove the pork gently from the sauce and transfer it to a board to rest for 10 minutes.

Meanwhile, place the cooking pan on the stovetop on low heat and very gently whisk the milk solids into the sauce. You don't need to completely break it up, as the ricotta-like clumps are completely delicious as they are. Taste and add more lemon juice and salt and pepper as desired, then add the remaining sage leaves and stir to wilt.

>

Place the pork on a serving platter and separate into pieces using tongs or a fork and spoon. Pour the sauce over and serve with a drizzle of olive oil.

Store in an airtight container in the refrigerator for up to 2 days, or freeze for up to 3 months.

For younger babies shred some of the pork and purée it with some of the juices until smooth. Serve with puréed vegies. Allow to cool before serving.

For older babies shred the meat for finger food and serve with finely chopped greens. Allow to cool before serving.

For toddlers serve as for adults, but allow to cool before serving.

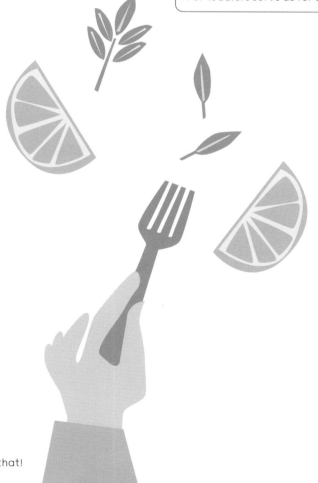

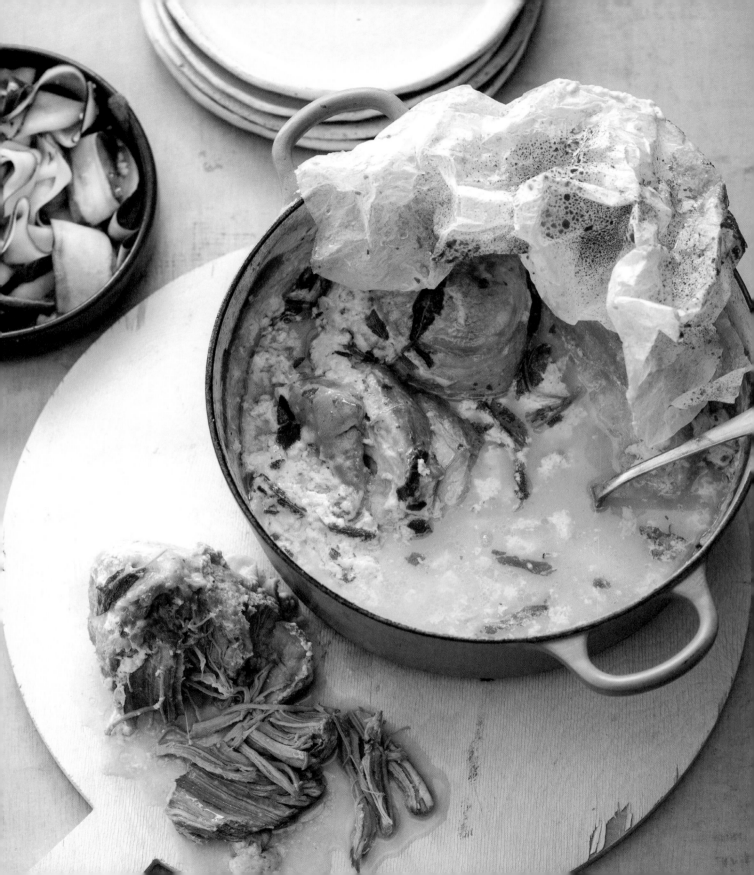

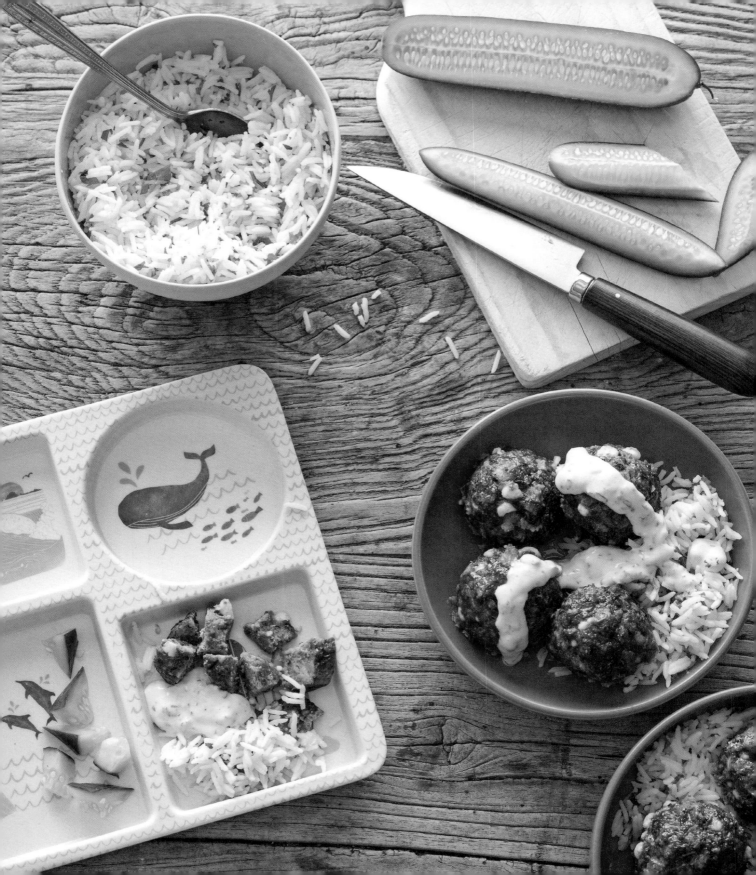

LAMB MEATBALLS WITH MINTED YOGHURT SAUCE

SERVES 4

PREP TIME: 15 MINUTES

COOKING TIME: 20 MINUTES

OPTIONAL

Kids of all ages love meatballs, and this recipe is easy, fragrant and flavourful. It's great as an appetiser or part of a light grazing lunch. Serve with some fresh cucumber, Pilaf (page 109), simple steamed rice, couscous salad or flatbread.

100 g (3½ oz) day-old bread, torn roughly into pieces

500 g (1 lb 2 oz) minced (ground) lamb

50 g (1¾ oz/⅓ cup) crumbled feta

40 g (1½ oz/¼ cup) macadamia nuts, finely chopped (optional)

1 small red onion, roughly chopped

1 garlic clove, crushed

1 tablespoon chopped flat-leaf (Italian) parsley

1 teaspoon ground coriander

1 teaspoon ground cumin

1 teaspoon dried oregano

½ teaspoon ground cinnamon

½ teaspoon sweet paprika

sea salt (omit for babies)

ground white pepper (just a tiny amount for babies)

MINTED YOGHURT SAUCE

250 g (9 oz/1 cup) Greek-style yoghurt

25 g (1 oz/½ cup) finely shredded mint leaves

1 garlic clove, crushed

juice of 1 lemon

¼ teaspoon ground cumin

¼ teaspoon cayenne pepper

sea salt (omit for babies)

ground white pepper (just a tiny amount for babies)

To make the minted yoghurt sauce, place the yoghurt, mint, garlic, lemon juice, cumin and cayenne in a small bowl and stir to combine. Let sit for 30 minutes before serving, to allow the flavours to develop. Season with salt and pepper to taste.

Preheat the oven to 180°C (350°F). Line a baking tray with baking paper.

Blitz the bread and macadamia nuts (if using) in a food processor to make crumbs.

Combine the remaining ingredients in a large mixing bowl, add the crumbs and mix well. Make sure the mixture is well seasoned. Roll into golf ball-sized balls and place on the lined tray. Bake in the oven for 20 minutes.

Store in an airtight container in the refrigerator for up to 2 days, or freeze for up to 3 months.

> **For younger babies** purée half a meatball in some minted yoghurt sauce until smooth - add a little water if it's too thick. Allow to cool before serving.
>
> **For older babies** shred the meatballs and serve as finger food with chopped cucumber and the minted yoghurt sauce. Allow to cool before serving.
>
> **For toddlers** serve as for adults, but allow to cool before serving.

POTATO-TOPPED FISH PIE

SERVES 6

PREP TIME: 35 MINUTES

COOKING TIME: 30 MINUTES

This recipe looks like a lot of work, but in fact is quite simple when you break it down into the three separate processes – mashed potato, the fish mixture and the white sauce. You can make extra mashed potato and put some aside for tomorrow's dinner. Likewise any left-over white sauce (béchamel). The fish pie requires nothing more to accompany it than a fresh green salad. You can make this recipe gluten-free by using gluten-free flour and brown rice crumbs instead of the breadcrumbs.

800 g (1 lb 12 oz) desiree or all-purpose potatoes

150 g (5½ oz) butter

150 ml (5 fl oz) full-cream (whole) milk

100 ml (3½ fl oz) pouring (single/light) cream

sea salt (omit for babies)

ground white pepper (just a tiny amount for babies)

3 tablespoons olive oil

1 leek, white part only, well washed and thinly sliced

3 garlic cloves, finely chopped (just a tiny amount for babies)

1.2 kg (2 lb 10 oz) white fish fillets, skinned and pin-boned, cut into large chunks

400 ml (13½ fl oz) quality fish or vegetable stock (preferably preservative and additive free)

125 ml (4 fl oz/½ cup) dry white wine

50 g (1¾ oz/⅓ cup) plain (all-purpose) flour (substitute gluten-free flour if family members are gluten-intolerant or coeliac)

1 tablespoon dijon mustard (just a tiny amount for babies)

handful of mixed herbs, such as chives, dill or tarragon, finely chopped

15 g (½ oz/¼ cup) panko (Japanese) breadcrumbs, or brown rice crumbs, mixed with 2 tablespoons melted butter

lemon wedges, to serve

To make the mashed potato for the top of your pie, steam or microwave the potatoes until tender. Set aside until cool enough to handle.

Combine one-third of the butter with half the milk and all the cream in a small saucepan and season with a good pinch of salt and pepper. Place over medium heat and bring to a gentle simmer. Remove from the heat and set aside in a warm place with the lid on.

Heat a large deep frying pan over medium heat with the olive oil and another third of the butter. When the butter has melted, add the leek and garlic with a pinch of salt and cook gently, without colouring, for about 4 minutes, stirring constantly, until the leek is soft. Add the fish, stock and wine and bring to a simmer. Simmer for about 4 minutes until the fish is just cooked through (this will also cook off the wine). Remove from the heat and scoop the fish and leek mixture into a colander to drain.

When the potatoes are cool enough to handle but still warm, peel them. (This is the only time I ever peel a potato, but it's OK if you don't!) Place the potatoes in a bowl and mash them as smoothly as you can. Add the warm milk mixture, stirring well but taking care not to overmix (don't do this in a food processor or the potatoes will be gluey). Set aside.

Pour the stock from the fish and the remaining milk into a small saucepan and bring to a simmer over medium heat. Reduce the heat to low.

To make a white sauce (or béchamel), place a medium saucepan over medium heat and melt the remaining butter. Slowly add the flour, stirring constantly for 2 minutes or until the paste just starts to toast around the edges. Now add the hot stock and milk mixture and keep stirring until a smooth, thick sauce forms. Add the mustard and herbs and season to taste with salt and pepper.

Preheat the oven to 160°C (320°F).

Add the fish and leek mixture to the sauce, stirring gently to combine. Transfer to a large pie dish and top with the mashed potato, using a fork to spread the potato over the dish. Sprinkle with the crumbs, then bake for 15–20 minutes, or until the filling is heated through and the topping is golden. Store in an airtight container in the refrigerator for up to 2 days, or freeze for up to 3 months.

For younger babies the pie is so soft you can mash it - or purée it - until smooth. Dilute with a little water if it's too thick. Allow to cool before serving.

For older babies mash the pie coarsely and serve with chopped cucumber and plain yoghurt. Allow to cool before serving.

For toddlers serve as for adults, but allow to cool before serving.

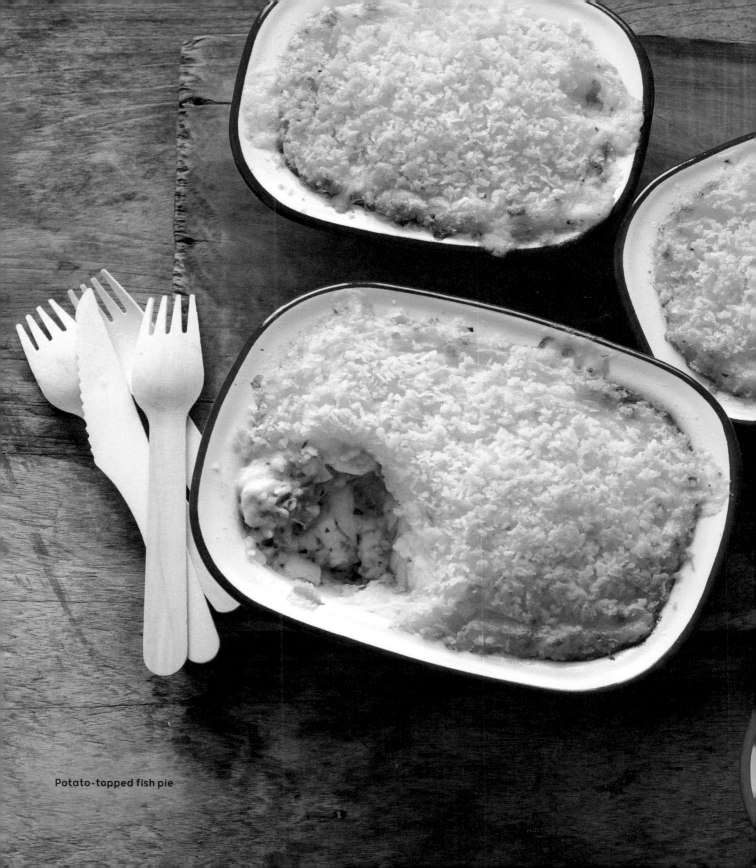

Potato-topped fish pie

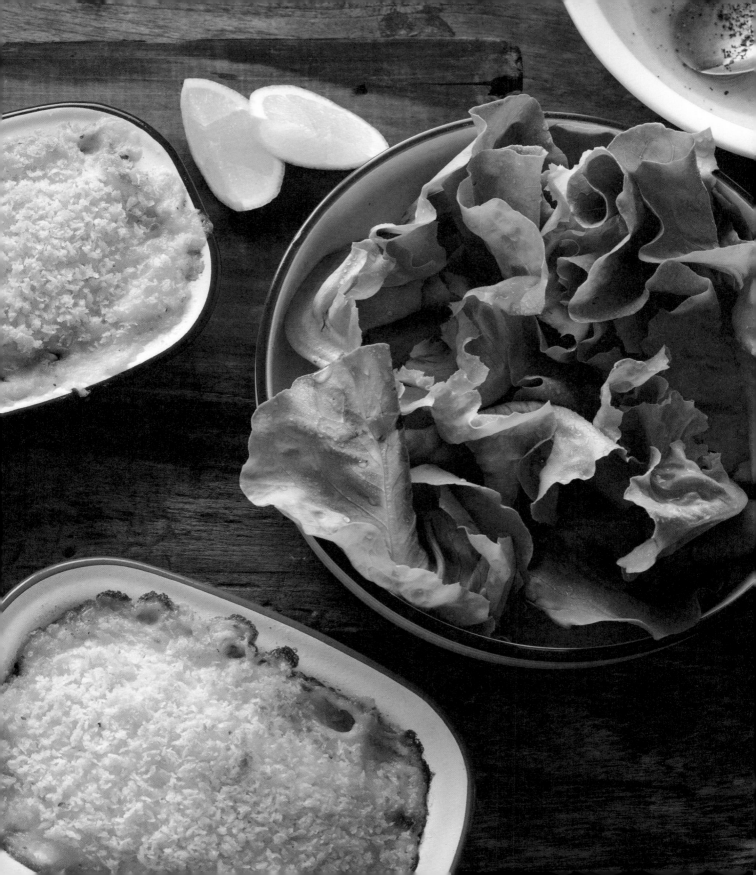

cakes, puddings and desserts

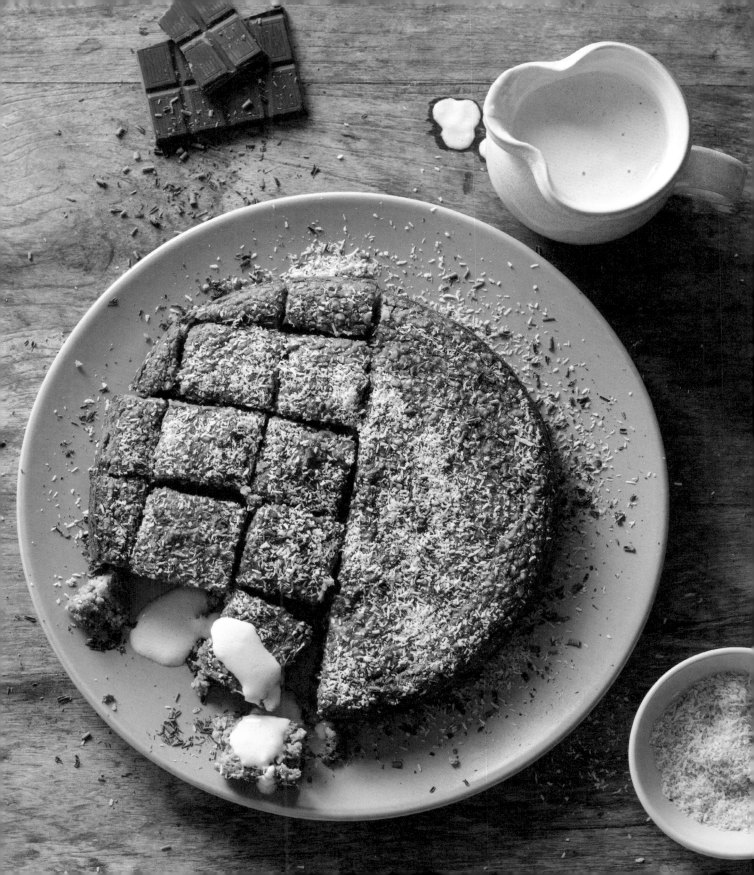

ORANGE AND ALMOND CAKE WITH TOASTED COCONUT

SERVES ABOUT 20

PREP TIME: 10 MINUTES

COOKING TIME: 3 HOURS

OPTIONAL

Packed full of protein and good fats, this flourless cake is always a winner. We've intentionally made the cake not too sweet. To add a touch more sweetness, serve it with a drizzle of Old-fashioned custard (page 189). Try making it with ground hazelnuts instead of the ground almonds, and for a special treat finish it with a little grated dark chocolate. You can cook the oranges a day or two before, to make things easy.

2 oranges (preferably organic or low-spray), skin on, washed thoroughly

3 eggs

105 g (3½ oz/¾ cup) coconut sugar

200 g (7 oz/2 cups) ground almonds

2 teaspoons baking powder

30 g (1 oz/⅓ cup) shredded or desiccated coconut, toasted, to serve

grated dark chocolate, to serve (optional)

Bring a large saucepan of water to the boil. Place the whole oranges gently in the water so they are fully immersed. Reduce the heat to medium and simmer for 2 hours - you may need to add extra water if it evaporates. Remove the oranges from the water and leave to cool to room temperature. When cold, place in a food processor and purée until smooth. The purée can be made a day or two ahead of time and kept in the refrigerator.

Preheat the oven to 160°C (320°F). Grease and line a 22 cm (8¾ in) springform cake tin with baking paper.

Beat the eggs and sugar with an electric mixer until well combined. Stir through the orange purée, ground almonds and baking powder. Pour the batter into the cake tin and bake for about 1-1¼ hours, until the top is golden and a skewer inserted into the centre comes out clean.

Allow the cake to cool in the tin before carefully removing. Serve sprinkled with toasted coconut and grated chocolate, if desired. Cut into squares or wedges. Store in an airtight container in the refrigerator for up to 3 days, or freeze for up to 3 months.

For younger babies purée a tiny amount of crumbled cake with a big dollop of custard for a special treat.

For older babies put a small amount of crumbled cake onto a big dollop of custard for a delicious dessert.

For toddlers serve as for adults.

PUMPKIN AND ALMOND SLICE

MAKES 24 PIECES

PREP TIME: 10 MINUTES

COOKING TIME: 50 MINUTES

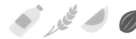

This is a delicious recipe for all ages, as a mid-morning coffee break or pick-me-up, and it's great in lunch boxes or as a first cake for older babies. We prefer to use butternut pumpkin (squash) for its natural sweetness, but it's fine to use a different variety.

½ butternut pumpkin (squash) – makes about 375 g (13 oz/1⅓ cups) mashed pumpkin

250 g (9 oz) butter, softened

230 g (8 oz/1 firmly packed cup) brown sugar

225 g (8 oz/1⅓ cups) plain (all-purpose) flour (substitute gluten-free flour if family members are gluten-intolerant or coeliac)

185 g (6½ oz/2 cups) quick oats

4 eggs, beaten

80 g (2¾ oz/⅓ cup) almonds (skin on), ground or very finely chopped

1 tablespoon maple syrup

1 teaspoon ground cinnamon

1 teaspoon ground ginger (just a tiny amount for babies)

½ teaspoon ground nutmeg (just a tiny amount for babies)

½ teaspoon salt (omit for babies)

Peel the pumpkin and cut it into chunks. Steam for 10 minutes, until the pumpkin can be easily pierced with a knife, then mash with a potato masher - don't purée, as you want to keep some texture.

Preheat the oven to 180°C (350°F). Line a 23 x 33 cm (8¾ x 13¼ in) shallow baking/slice tin.

Whisk the butter and brown sugar using an electric mixer until light and creamy. Stir in the flour and oats. Add the egg to the mixture, along with the mashed pumpkin and remaining ingredients. Mix gently for another 15 seconds or until just combined.

Pour the mixture into the tin (the mixture should be about 2 cm/¾ in deep), then bake for 40 minutes. When cooked it should be lightly browned and a skewer inserted into the slice should come out clean.

Allow to cool on a wire rack. Serve cut into squares.

Store in an airtight container in the refrigerator for up to 3 days, or freeze for up to 3 months.

> **For younger babies 7 months plus** who can chew or gum their food, this is a lovely soft, smooth slice.
>
> **For older babies** break off small pieces of the slice to serve.
>
> **For toddlers** serve as for adults.

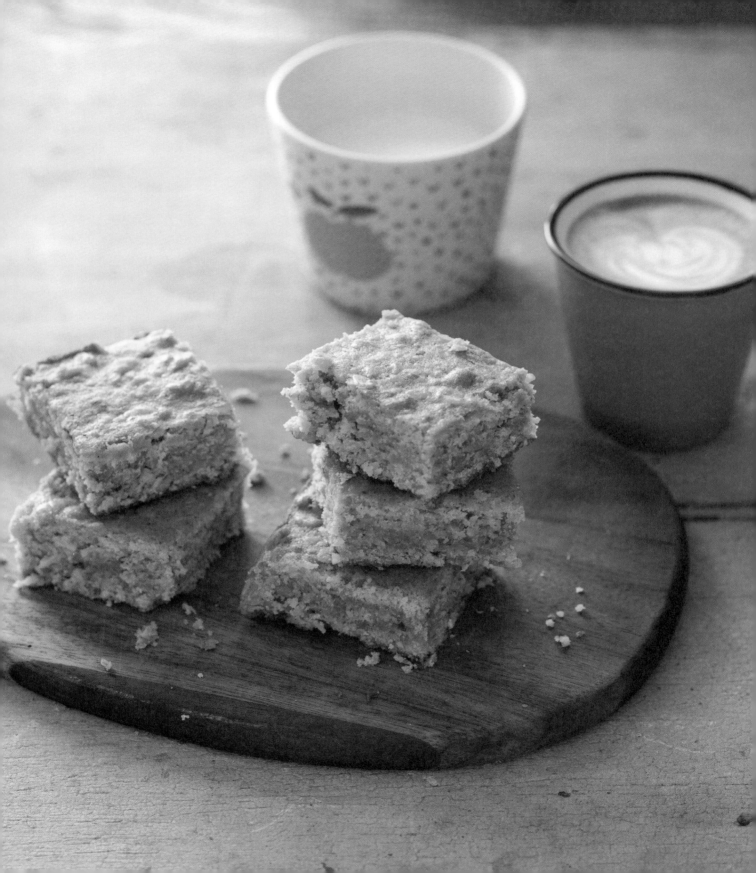

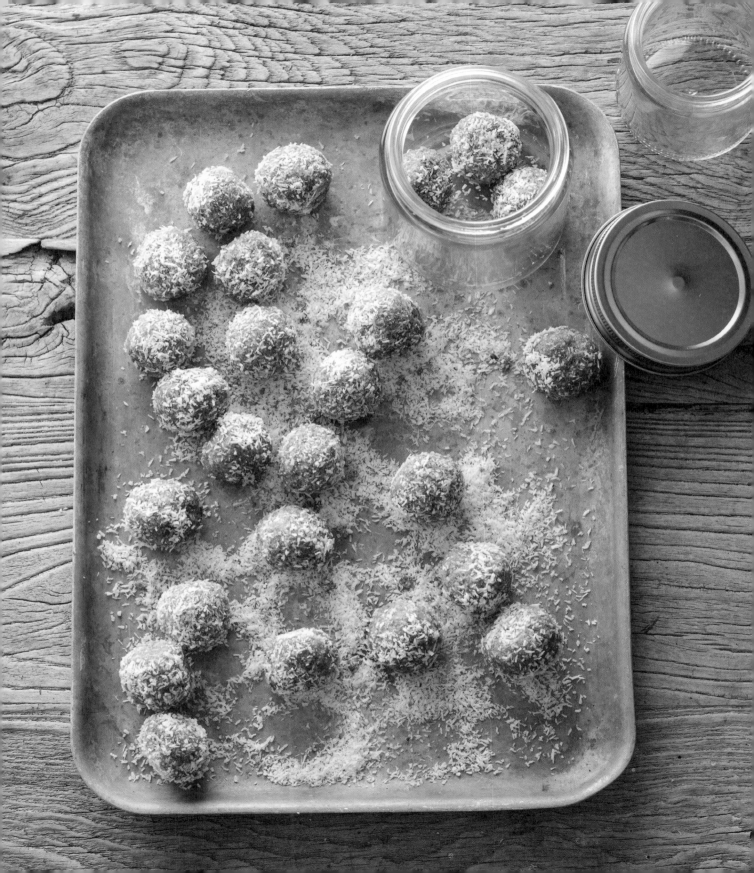

COCONUT MACADAMIA ENERGY BALLS

MAKES 12 BALLS (OR MORE IF SMALLER)

PREP TIME: 10 MINUTES, PLUS CHILLING

A quick and easy no-bake recipe, these are the ultimate grab and go treat. They can be frozen and also dropped into smoothies as a protein-rich, naturally sweet bomb.

310 g (11 oz/2 cups) almonds, skin on

80 g (2¾ oz/½ cup) macadamia nuts

125 g (4½ oz/1 cup) sultanas (golden raisins)

185 g (6½ oz/¼ cup) goji berries

1 teaspoon natural vanilla extract

1 teaspoon ground cinnamon (use a tiny amount for young babies)

3 tablespoons melted coconut oil

45 g (1½ oz/½ cup) desiccated coconut, for rolling

Combine the nuts, sultanas, goji berries, vanilla and cinnamon in a food processor and blitz well until smooth, adding the coconut oil to bring it all together.

Transfer the mixture to a bowl and roll it into balls about 3 cm (1¼ in) in diameter, using your hands or a melon baller.

Spread the desiccated coconut in a shallow bowl, then roll the balls in the coconut until evenly coated. Chill in the refrigerator for a few hours.

Store in an airtight container in the refrigerator for up to 3 days, or freeze for up to 3 months.

> **For younger babies 7 months plus** who are ready for some finger food, tear into squishy finger food-sized pieces.
>
> **For older babies** tear into squishy finger food-sized pieces.
>
> **For toddlers** serve as for adults.

BLACK STICKY RICE WITH COCONUT AND MANGO

SERVES 6

PREP TIME: 5 MINUTES

COOKING TIME: 10 MINUTES, PLUS RESTING

OPTIONAL

Black sticky rice is a staple throughout Southeast Asia. Its sweet, earthy flavour makes for a nourishing breakfast or dessert. This nutritious dish can grow up to be a dinner-party favourite, served with coconut ice cream or a lemon sorbet.

350 g (12½ oz/1¾ cups) black rice
90 g (3 oz/¼ cup) ground dark palm sugar (jaggery)
500 ml (17 fl oz/2 cups) coconut milk
125 ml (4 fl oz/½ cup) coconut cream
1 large ripe mango, peeled and cut into wedges or thinly sliced
maple syrup
2 tablespoons desiccated coconut, lightly toasted
1 tablespoon smooth, unsalted peanut butter (see Home-made nut butters on page 217) (optional)

Place the rice in a fine-mesh sieve and rinse it well in cold water. Drain.

Transfer the rice to a medium saucepan with the palm sugar and 750 ml (25½ fl oz/3 cups) water and bring to the boil. Reduce the heat to medium-low and simmer for about 10 minutes, or until the water is absorbed. Remove from the heat, place a tight-fitting lid on the pan and set aside for 40 minutes to allow the rice to finish cooking with the residual heat and steam. Add the coconut milk to the rice and stir through. (Set aside baby's and toddler's portions now.)

To serve, spoon the rice into bowls and top each with a spoon of coconut cream, some mango wedges, a drizzle of maple syrup and some toasted coconut. Add a dollop of peanut butter, if desired.

Store in an airtight container in the refrigerator for up to 2 days, or freeze for up to 3 months.

> **For younger babies** purée the sticky rice until smooth - add a little extra coconut milk to dilute it if it's too thick. Top with a little smooth, unsalted peanut butter and mango purée, if desired. Allow to cool before serving.
>
> **For older babies** top the sticky rice with some soft mango chunks and coconut cream. Allow to cool before serving.
>
> **For toddlers** serve as for adults, but allow to cool before serving.

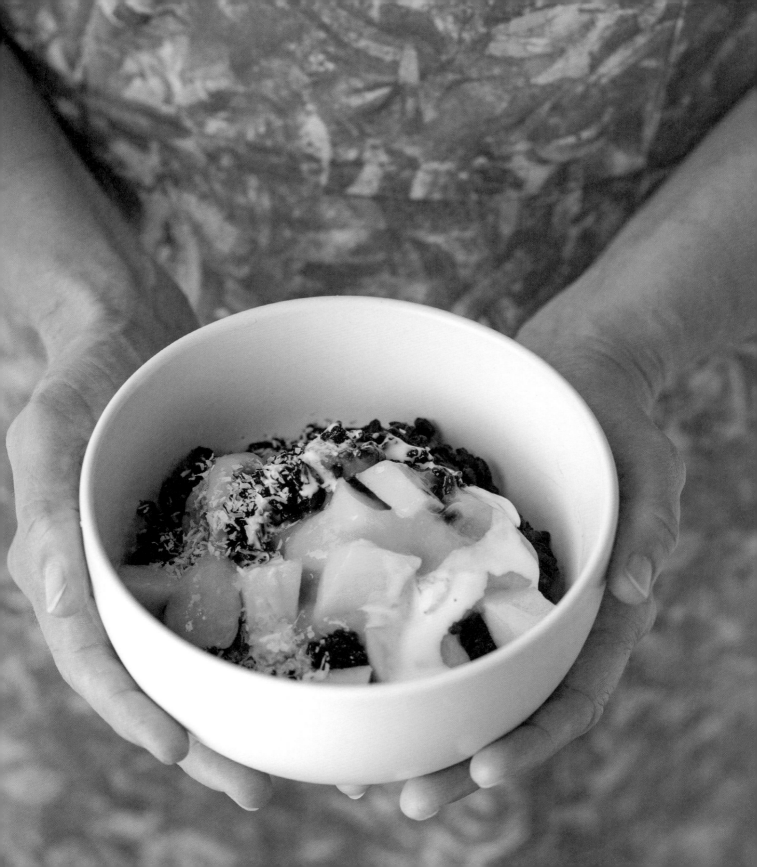

COCONUT RICE PUDDING

OPTIONAL

This is such a nourishing and sustaining little pudding, ideal for any time of day, but especially as a dessert, and it's made in a flash.

500 ml (17 fl oz/2 cups) coconut milk
370 g (13 oz/2 cups) cooked brown rice
2 tablespoons maple syrup
2 teaspoons smooth, unsalted, macadamia butter or peanut butter (see Home-made nut butters on page 217)
ground cinnamon, to serve (optional)

Add the coconut milk to a medium saucepan and bring gently to a simmer. Add the rice, maple syrup and macadamia butter and mix well to combine. Continue to simmer over low heat for 5 minutes or until thickened. Serve with a sprinkling of cinnamon, if desired.

Store in an airtight container in the refrigerator for up to 2 days, or freeze for up to 3 months.

> **For younger babies** omit the cinnamon sprinkle. Purée until smooth. Allow to cool before serving.
>
> **For older babies** keep the serving size small and accompany with a fruit purée. Allow to cool before serving.
>
> **For toddlers** serve as for adults, but allow to cool before serving.

CHIA PUDDING WITH BERRIES, YOGHURT AND MACADAMIA

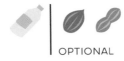

OPTIONAL

This is so easy to prepare and makes a delicious creamy, tangy and slightly sweet dessert. Chia seeds are rich in omega-3 fatty acids. Be sure to always soak them for at least 30 minutes. If not soaked sufficiently, the seeds can expand within the throat or gut, increasing the risk of choking or indigestion. This also makes a great breakfast – prepare the pudding the night before, then serve with the yoghurt and macadamia sprinkle.

95 g (3¼ oz/½ cup) chia seeds (black or white)
500 ml (17 fl oz/2 cups) coconut water
350 g (12¼ oz) mixed fresh berries
2 tablespoons maple syrup
2 teaspoons natural vanilla extract
grated zest and juice of 1 lemon
500 g (1 lb 2 oz/2 cups) Greek-style yoghurt
2 tablespoons raw macadamia nuts, crushed or finely chopped (or smooth macadamia butter for babies, see Home-made nut butters on page 217), to serve (optional)

Soak the chia seeds in the coconut water for at least 30 minutes (this is important). Meanwhile, combine half the berries with the maple syrup, vanilla, lemon zest and juice and allow to steep for 20 minutes.

Add the berry mixture to the soaked chia seeds and stir well to combine.

Spoon the chia-berry mixture into the base of four individual serving glasses. Add a layer of yoghurt followed by a layer of fresh berries, to create a trifle effect. Finish with the crushed macadamia nuts.

Store in an airtight container in the refrigerator for up to 3 days.

> **For younger babies** purée the chia-berry mixture until smooth. Top with a dollop of smooth macadamia butter.
>
> **For older babies** mash any lumpy fruits and serve as is with a dollop of smooth macadamia butter or finely ground macadamia nuts.
>
> **For toddlers** serve as for adults, but ensure that any nuts are finely chopped.

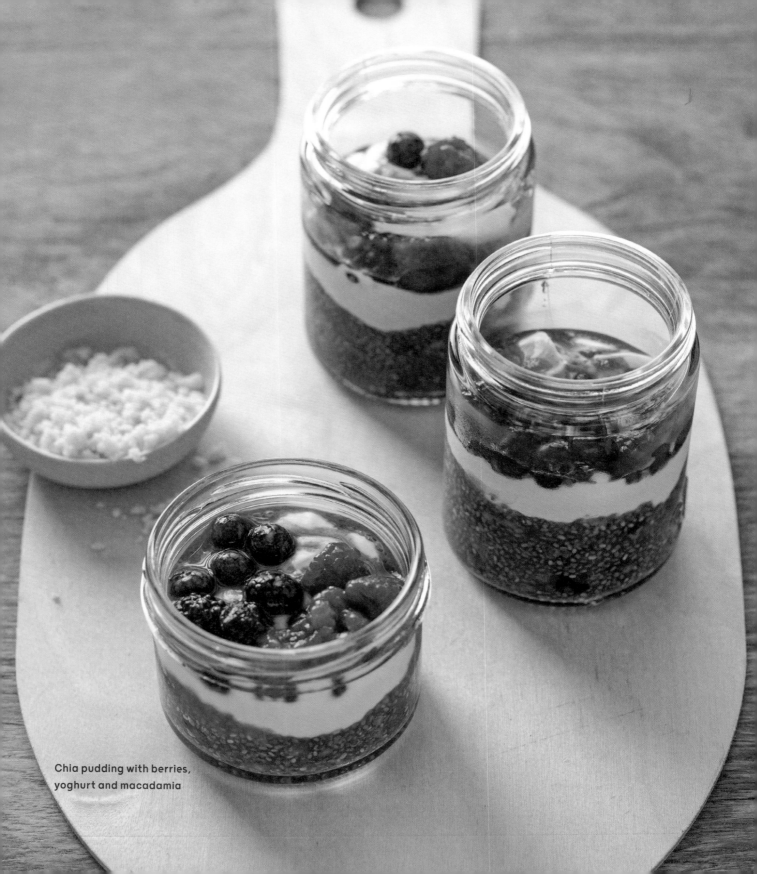

Chia pudding with berries, yoghurt and macadamia

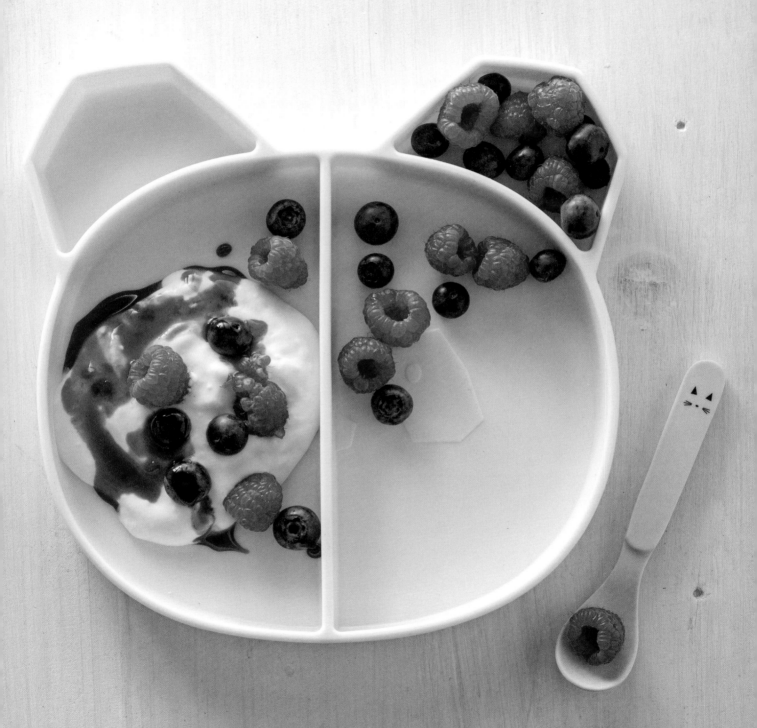

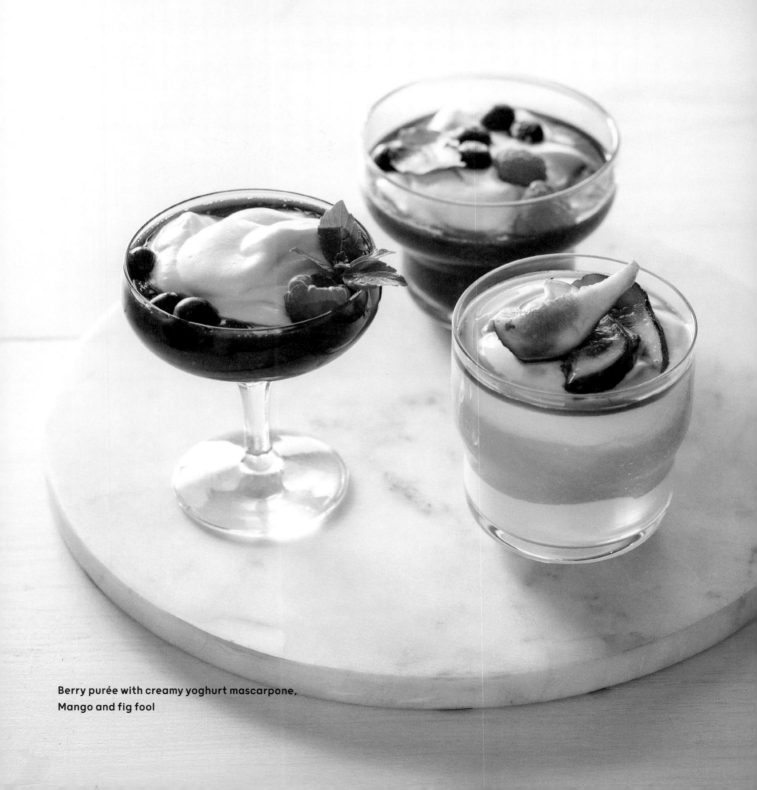

Berry purée with creamy yoghurt mascarpone,
Mango and fig fool

MANGO AND FIG FOOL

SERVES 4

PREP TIME: 5 MINUTES, PLUS RESTING

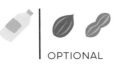

OPTIONAL

Fruit fools are a simple dessert that can be put together in no time. Ours is a healthier, less sweet and less rich twist on the traditional version – we've cut out the cream and sugar but kept all the flavour. Instead of mango and fig, you can use strawberries, raspberries, blackberries or blueberries, or try mango pulp and passionfruit finished with some toasted coconut flakes. (Frozen pulps are a further time-saver.) Instead of yoghurt, try using smooth creamy cottage cheese, then fold ground almonds or hazelnuts or very finely crushed pistachio nuts through the fool.

2 ripe mangoes
1 teaspoon natural vanilla extract
500 g (1 lb 2 oz/2 cups) Greek-style yoghurt or full-fat plain yoghurt
1 tablespoon maple syrup
2 figs, thinly sliced or cut into wedges

Peel the mangoes and cut the flesh off the seeds. Purée the flesh using a hand-held blender. Set aside.

Add the vanilla to the yoghurt and mix it through. Chill in the refrigerator for 15 minutes.

To serve, spoon a layer of the yoghurt into individual serving glasses, followed by some mango purée. Add more yoghurt and a drizzle of maple syrup. Top with the sliced fig.

Store in an airtight container in the refrigerator for up to 24 hours.

> **For younger babies** leave out the fig and serve as is.
>
> **For older babies** top the fool with finely chopped fig.
>
> **For toddlers** serve as for adults.

BERRY PURÉE WITH CREAMY YOGHURT MASCARPONE

SERVES 4

PREP TIME: 15 MINUTES

COOKING TIME: 5 MINUTES

This is easy to prepare and perfect for a special dinner, and the bonus is that it's healthy. The berry purée is great used as a jam on toast or pikelets.

220 g (8 oz/1 cup) mascarpone
250 g (9 oz/1 cup) Greek-style yoghurt
1 teaspoon natural vanilla extract
1 tablespoon maple syrup
mint sprigs, to garnish

BERRY PURÉE
350 g (12¼ oz) mixed berries, fresh
    or frozen
60 g (2 oz) caster (superfine) sugar
juice of ½ lemon

To make the berry purée, place two-thirds of the berries in a medium saucepan with the sugar and lemon juice. Bring gently to the boil over medium heat, then reduce the heat to medium-low and simmer for about 4 minutes, until the sugar has dissolved and the berries are just starting to collapse. Remove from the heat and set aside to cool. When cool, purée in a blender.

Beat the mascarpone using an electric mixer. When it gets to soft peaks add the yoghurt, vanilla and maple syrup and whip on medium speed until thick and creamy.

Pour the berry purée into martini glasses and top with a big dollop of the mascarpone mixture. Serve the remaining berries on top with a sprig of mint.

Store in an airtight container in the refrigerator for up to 24 hours.

> **For younger and older babies** serve without the additional berries or mint on top.
>
> **For toddlers** serve as for adults, with plenty of mascarpone.

OLD-FASHIONED CUSTARD

MAKES 500 G
(1 LB 2 OZ/2¼ CUPS)

PREP TIME: 3 MINUTES

COOKING TIME: 7 MINUTES

Custard is making a comeback and rightly so, as it's delicious, rich in protein and easy to digest. Serve with poached fruit, cakes or puddings.

500 ml (17 fl oz/2 cups) milk
1 teaspoon natural vanilla extract
2 eggs, plus 2 egg yolks
1 tablespoon maple syrup

Heat the milk and vanilla in a medium saucepan on medium heat until warmed through. Remove from the heat and set aside. Combine the whole eggs, egg yolks and maple syrup in a bowl and whisk using an electric mixer until smooth and creamy (1–2 minutes). Slowly pour in the warm milk, continuing to whisk until combined. Return the mixture to the saucepan and, over low heat, whisk constantly until the mixture starts to thicken, coating the back of a spoon. Remove from the heat and whisk for another 30 seconds. Pour the custard into a jug and allow to cool. Store in an airtight container in the refrigerator for up to 3 days.

> **For younger babies** serve as is or with a fruit purée.
>
> **For older babies** serve as is or with mashed fresh or stewed fruits.
>
> **For toddlers** serve as for adults.

Variation

MAKES ABOUT 840 G
(1 LB 14 OZ/3–3¼ CUPS)

BANANA CUSTARD

To make a banana-flavoured, stand-alone dessert, omit the maple syrup in the recipe above and simply add 3 peeled and finely chopped bananas at the point where you remove the custard from the heat. Purée using a hand-held blender until smooth. Store in an airtight container in the refrigerator for up to 3 days.

> **For younger babies** serve as is.
>
> **For older babies** serve as is or with additional mashed fresh or stewed fruits.
>
> **For toddlers** serve as for adults.

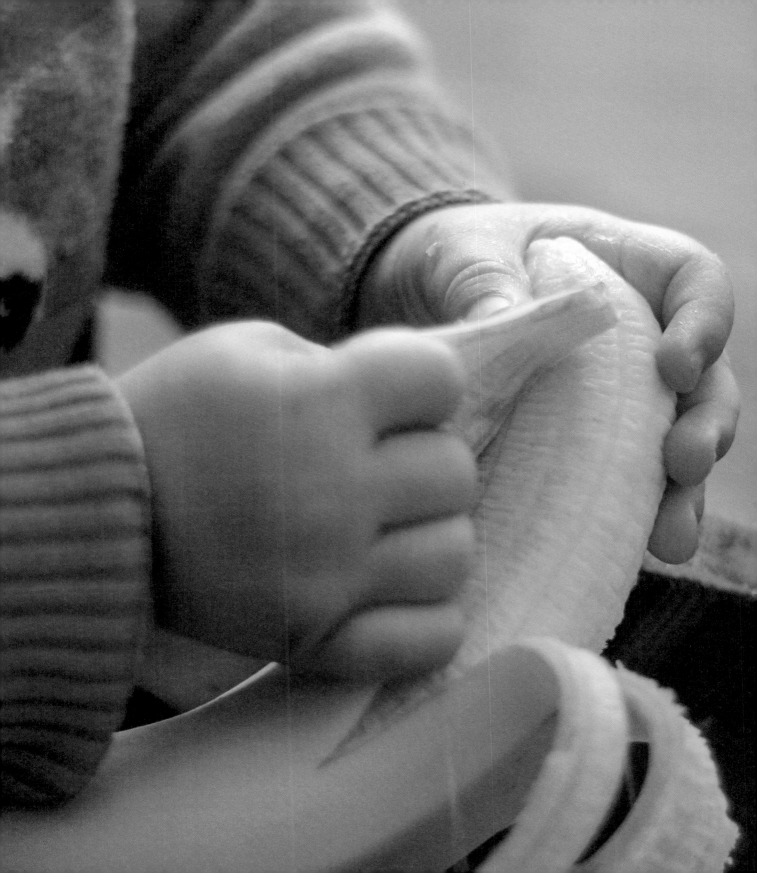

BANANA BREAD

MAKES 1 LOAF

PREP TIME: 5 MINUTES

COOKING TIME: 60 MINUTES

Bananas are usually always available and relatively affordable, so a good banana bread is a must in any cook's repertoire and is a great way to use softer bananas. Deliciously moist and not too sweet, this will become a family favourite, and it's so easy you don't need to be a baker to make it. Bring out the banana bread when visitors come over for morning or afternoon tea.

3 ripe bananas, peeled and roughly chopped

190 g (6¾ oz/1¾ cups) mixed nut meal (almond, hazelnut, macadamia)

150 g (5¼ oz/1 cup) quality plain (all-purpose) flour (substitute a quality gluten-free flour if family members are gluten-intolerant or coeliac)

55 g (2 oz/firmly packed ¼ cup) brown sugar

2 eggs

3 tablespoons maple syrup

3 tablespoons coconut oil, melted

2 teaspoons baking powder

1 teaspoon natural vanilla extract

¼ teaspoon ground cinnamon (just a tiny amount for babies)

pinch of sea salt (omit for babies)

Preheat the oven to 160°C (320°F). Line a 25 x 10.5 x 7 cm (10 x 4¼ x 2¾ in) loaf (bar) tin with baking paper.

Place all the ingredients in an electric mixer and blitz for about 90 seconds until there are no large lumps, but do not purée. Bake in the oven for 1-1¼ hours, until the surface is a rich brown colour and a skewer comes out clean when inserted into the bread.

Let the bread cool in the tin on a wire rack, then remove from the tin and allow to cool completely before slicing.

Store in an airtight container in the refrigerator for up to 2 days, or freeze for up to 3 months.

> **For younger babies** wait until after 7 months when your baby is ready for their first finger foods, then serve small pieces.
>
> **For older babies and toddlers** banana bread makes fabulous finger food.

dips,
dressings
and sauces

GUACAMOLE

MAKES 480 G (1 LB 1 OZ/2 CUPS)

PREP TIME: 5 MINUTES

This guacamole is so easy to make at home. Rich in monounsaturated fats and gut-friendly fibre, avocados are always popular with the whole family. The squeeze of lime cuts through the rich avocado to make the dip refreshing and delicious. This is a must with Sweet corn and macadamia fritters (page 80), or serve it as a dip with grissini or fresh vegies cut into sticks.

OPTIONAL

2 tablespoons finely chopped red onion
sea salt (omit for babies)
small handful of roughly chopped coriander (cilantro) leaves
2 ripe avocados, pitted and peeled
juice of 1 lime
jalapeño, minced (omit for babies)
freshly ground black pepper (just a tiny amount for babies)
grissini, to serve (optional)

If you have a large mortar and pestle this is fun to make using it (otherwise use a food processor). Place the onion in the mortar with the salt and half the coriander and pound to a rough paste. Add the avocado and remaining coriander. Mash with a fork, then add the lime juice. At this point you can put some guacamole aside for small people while you spice up the remainder with jalapeño. Season to taste with salt and pepper.

Store in a sealed container in the refrigerator for up to 24 hours.

> **For younger babies** avocado is rich in fats so a suitable serving of this dish is about 2-3 teaspoons, and you can just serve it on its own. It's also perfect puréed with Sweet corn and macadamia fritters (page 80) until smooth.
>
> **For older babies** keep servings small. For babies ready for finger food, serve as a dip with toast 'soldiers' (finger-sized pieces).
>
> **For toddlers** serve as for adults, with grissini or toast fingers, if desired.

TZATZIKI

**MAKES ABOUT 345 G
(12 OZ/1¼ CUPS)**

**PREP TIME: 10 MINUTES,
PLUS CHILLING**

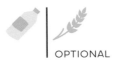

OPTIONAL

Refreshing tzatziki is a favourite in the summer months and makes a great accompaniment to most cooked meats and fish. It's also delicious with crudités and crackers. We love swapping the mint for dill in this recipe.

1 Lebanese (long) cucumber, split, deseeded and grated (about 110 g/ 4 oz/½ packed cup)
250 g (9 oz/1 cup) Greek-style yoghurt
¼ teaspoon crushed garlic (optional for babies)
1 tablespoon lemon juice
1 tablespoon finely chopped mint
sea salt (omit for babies)
freshly ground black pepper (just a tiny amount for babies)

Place the grated cucumber in a bowl lined with a clean tea towel (dish towel) or a piece of clean muslin (cheesecloth). Gather up the edges of the towel and squeeze to ring out the excess moisture from the cucumber. Set the cucumber aside.

In a large bowl, combine the yoghurt, garlic, lemon juice and mint. Add the cucumber and season with salt and pepper to taste. Cover and chill for at least 30 minutes, or ideally overnight, before serving.

Store in a sealed container in the refrigerator for up to 5 days.

> **For younger babies** purée to a silky smooth consistency. You can reduce or remove the garlic if the flavours are too strong for your baby.
>
> **For older babies** serve with pita bread fingers - purée the tzatziki if the cucumber is too chunky.
>
> **For toddlers** this makes a great dipping sauce to go with shredded chicken or other meats.

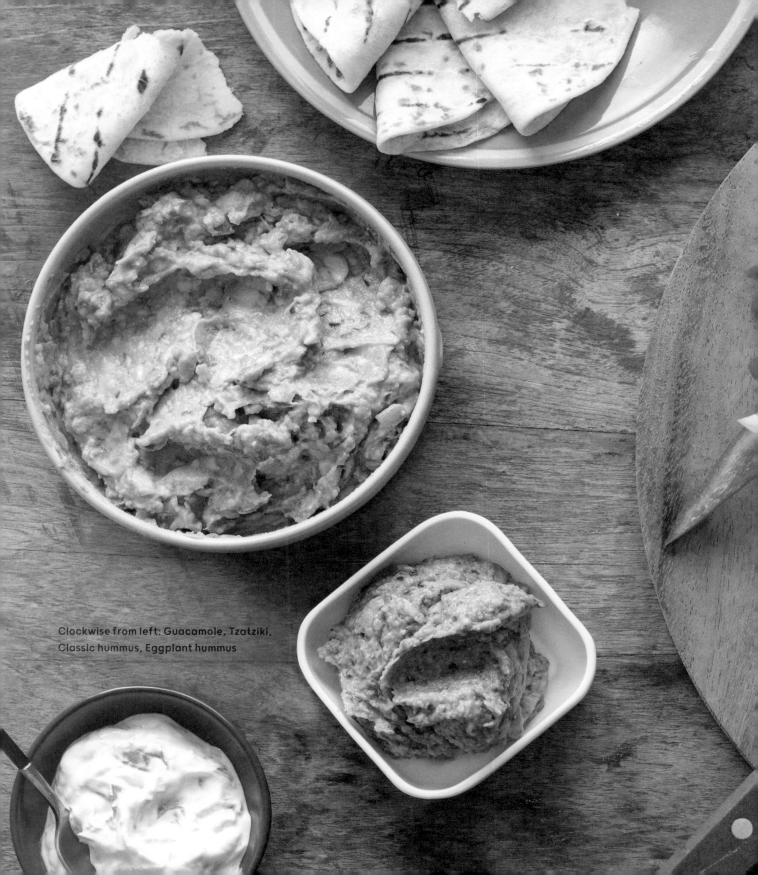

Clockwise from left: Guacamole, Tzatziki, Classic hummus, Eggplant hummus

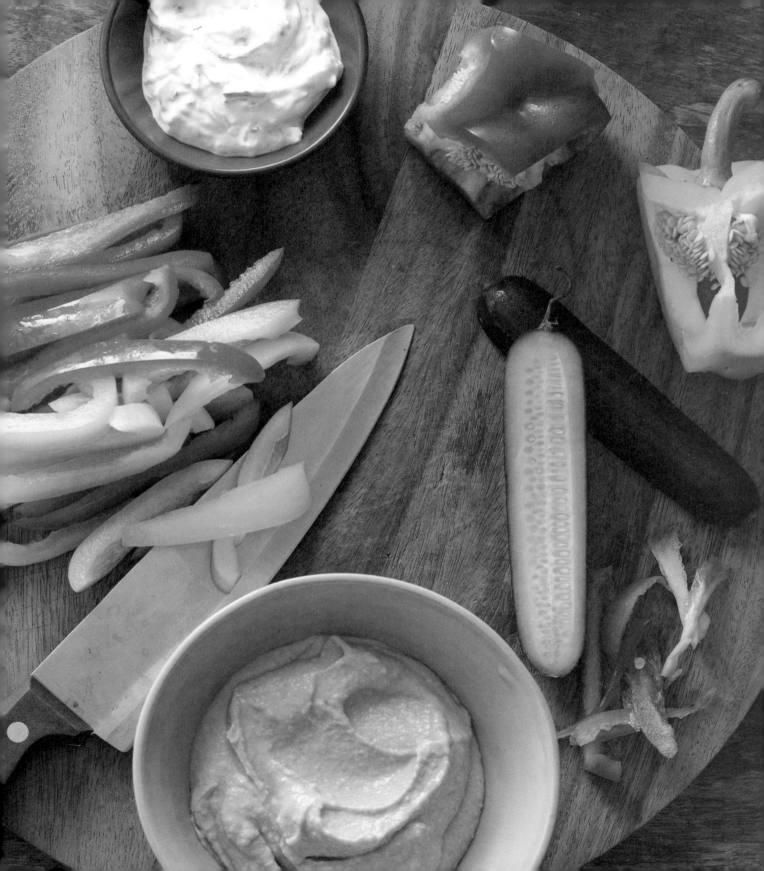

CLASSIC HUMMUS

**MAKES ABOUT 500 G
(1 LB 2 OZ/2 CUPS)**

PREP TIME: 5 MINUTES

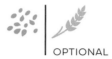

OPTIONAL

Chickpeas are rich in fibre and protein, and hummus makes for the perfect snack any time, as a spread or as a dip with crackers, celery and carrot sticks. The tahini in hummus is made from ground sesame seeds.

400 g (14 oz) tinned chickpeas, drained, liquid reserved
juice of 1 lemon
2 tablespoons hulled white tahini
½ teaspoon ground cumin
1 garlic clove, roughly chopped (optional for babies)
¼ teaspoon smoked paprika, plus extra to serve (just a tiny amount for babies)
3 tablespoons olive oil, plus extra to serve
¼ teaspoon sea salt (omit for babies)
¼ teaspoon freshly ground black pepper (less for babies)

In a food processor, pulse the chickpeas, lemon juice, tahini, cumin, garlic and smoked paprika until smooth. With the motor running, slowly pour in the oil in a steady stream. Purée until very smooth and creamy. If the mixture is too thick, add some of the reserved chickpea liquid, a little at a time. Season to taste.

To serve, sprinkle with extra smoked paprika and a drizzle of olive oil.

Store in a sealed container in the refrigerator for up to 2 days.

> **For younger babies** you can leave out the garlic to make a really mild hummus.
>
> **For older babies** this is great to serve as a spread on toast 'soldiers' (finger-sized pieces).
>
> **For toddlers** serve with celery or carrot sticks for dipping.

EGGPLANT HUMMUS

**MAKES ABOUT 700 G
(1 LB 9 OZ/2¾ CUPS)**

PREP TIME: 10 MINUTES

COOKING TIME: 45 MINUTES

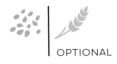

OPTIONAL

Technically not a traditional hummus, this version is light yet full-flavoured, and made with roasted eggplant and garlic.

2 medium eggplants (aubergines)
2 garlic cloves (optional for babies)
400 g (14 oz) tinned chickpeas, rinsed
    and drained
juice of 1 lemon
2 tablespoons white tahini
2 tablespoons flat-leaf (Italian) parsley
    leaves
2 tablespoons olive oil
sea salt (omit for babies)
freshly ground black pepper (just a tiny
    amount for babies)

Preheat the oven to 180°C (350°F).

Place the eggplants on a small baking tray and prick them all over with a fork. Roast for about 30 minutes, then add the garlic and cook for a further 10-15 minutes or until the eggplant is soft. Remove from the oven and allow to cool.

Remove the stalks from the eggplant and place the eggplant and garlic in the bowl of a food processor with the remaining ingredients. We like to leave the skin on the eggplant, but by all means remove it before blending if you prefer. Blend until well combined but still with a little texture. Season to taste.

Store in a sealed container in the refrigerator for up to 2 days.

> **For younger babies** purée to a silky smooth consistency. You may want to reduce or leave out the garlic if the flavour is too strong for your baby.
>
> **For older babies** this makes a delicious purée perfect to serve as a spread with toast 'soldiers' (finger-sized pieces).
>
> **For toddlers** serve with celery or carrot sticks for dipping.

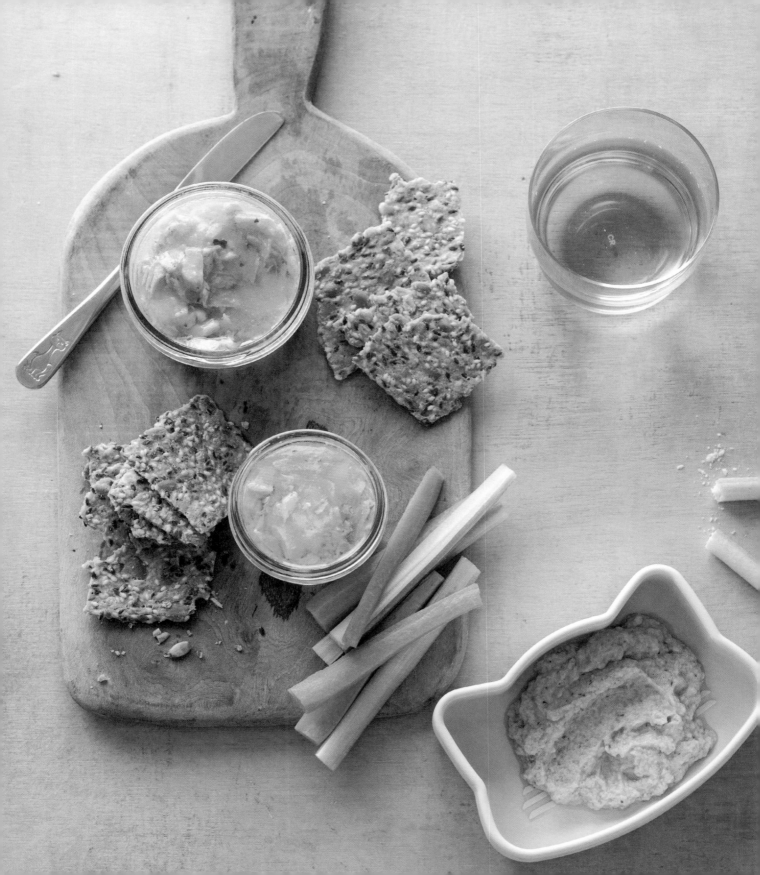

SALMON AND TARRAGON DIP

MAKES 600 G (1 LB 5 OZ/2 CUPS)

PREP TIME: 10 MINUTES,
PLUS CHILLING

COOKING TIME: 15 MINUTES

A simple salmon dip with fresh flavours that all the family will love. It's quick to whip up for impressive pre-dinner snacks, served with crudités, seed crackers or grissini.

OPTIONAL

400 g (14 oz) skinless salmon fillet, skinned, pin-boned and cut into large pieces
40 g (1¼ oz) unsalted butter
⅛ small red onion, finely diced
sea salt (omit for babies)
1 tablespoon crème fraîche or sour cream
1 tablespoon mascarpone
1 tablespoon finely chopped tarragon
1 tablespoon lemon juice
1 tablespoon olive oil
1 hard-boiled egg, finely minced or puréed to a paste
ground white pepper (just a tiny amount for babies)
ghee, to store

Bring a saucepan of water fitted with a steaming basket to the boil. Place the salmon on a plate that will fit in the basket, then place the plate in the steamer. Steam until just cooked but still pink in the centre, about 7-8 minutes. Remove the salmon from the steamer and set aside to cool.

Melt the butter in a frying pan over low heat. Add the onion with a tiny pinch of salt and cook until soft, about 4 minutes. Remove from the pan and allow to cool.

In a medium bowl, beat the crème fraîche, mascarpone and tarragon together with a wooden spoon until smooth. Add the cooked onion, lemon juice, olive oil and egg and stir thoroughly. Flake the salmon into the bowl and mix until well combined. Season to taste with salt and pepper. Chill for at least an hour before serving.

To store, place in a clean airtight container and cover with a layer of ghee. Refrigerate for up to 3 days.

For younger babies ensure the egg is well cooked. Purée everything until silky smooth.

For older babies ensure the egg is well cooked. Serve as a smooth purée, or slightly more chunky, with toast 'soldiers' (finger-sized pieces) or pita bread for dipping.

For toddlers serve as a coarse purée with vegetable sticks for dipping, or serve as for adults.

BASIL PESTO

MAKES 300 G (10¼ OZ/2 CUPS)

PREP TIME: 5 MINUTES

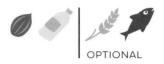

OPTIONAL

Pestos are flavour-packed and provide plenty of nutrients – mostly good fats and refreshing herbs. You can serve pesto with pasta, add a spoonful to soups and stews, or jazz up a sandwich – a teaspoon of pesto goes a very long way. Carrot-top pesto is a favourite variation of ours and uses the green carrot tops that might otherwise end up in the compost heap. Make sure they are really well washed and substitute carrot tops for all or half the basil. For another variation, you can do the same with coriander (cilantro) and rocket (arugula). Pesto is the building block for a great Green eggs and ham (page 77).

1 bunch basil, leaves only, rinsed and patted dry

1 garlic clove (optional for babies)

2 tablespoons pine nuts

3 tablespoons grated parmesan (use ricotta for babies)

250 ml (8½ fl oz/1 cup) extra virgin olive oil

sea salt (omit for babies)

freshly ground black pepper (just a tiny amount for babies)

Place the basil, garlic and pine nuts in a food processor and blend to a rough paste. Transfer to a bowl and stir through the parmesan and olive oil - enough to create a runny paste that still holds together well. Season to taste with salt and pepper.

Store in a sealed container in the refrigerator for up to 3 days.

For younger babies you might want to omit or reduce the garlic for babies, or add a dollop of natural yoghurt to make the flavour milder. Purée to a silky smooth consistency.

For older babies add a dollop of pesto to thoroughly cooked scrambled eggs.

For toddlers serve as for adults.

MINT AND ALMOND PESTO

MAKES 150 G (5¼ OZ/1 CUP)

PREP TIME: 5 MINUTES

Pesto is also wonderful when you swap the basil for mint and the pine nuts for almonds. Try this lively pesto with lamb, pasta, vegetables and seafood.

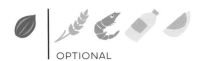

OPTIONAL

80 g (2¾ oz/4 lightly packed cups) mint leaves, rinsed and patted dry
80 ml (2½ fl oz/⅓ cup) olive oil, plus extra as required
50 g (1¾ oz/⅓ cup) blanched almonds, skin off
2 garlic cloves, roughly chopped (just a tiny amount for babies)
grated zest of 1 lemon
sea salt (omit for babies)
freshly ground black pepper (just a tiny amount for babies)

Blend all the ingredients together in a food processor, adding extra oil as required. Season to taste with salt and pepper.

For younger babies you can omit or reduce the amount of garlic in the recipe, and add some yoghurt or ricotta to lighten the flavour. Purée to a silky smooth consistency.

For older babies add a dollop of pesto to thoroughly cooked scrambled eggs.

For toddlers serve as for adults.

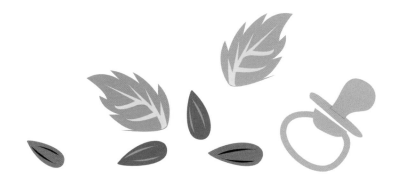

GREEN GODDESS AVOCADO DRESSING

This is our variation on the ultimate go-to dressing – delicious, fresh, simple and great on just about everything. Serve with seafood, as a salad dressing, a sandwich binder, or a great dipping sauce for vegetables and boiled eggs.

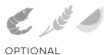

OPTIONAL

1 small red Asian shallot, roughly chopped
1 small garlic clove (just a tiny amount for babies)
1 tablespoon lime juice
1 tablespoon lemon juice
flesh of 1 avocado
handful of coriander (cilantro) leaves, washed, dried and roughly chopped
15 g (½ oz/½ cup) basil leaves, washed, dried and roughly chopped
25 g (1 oz/½ cup) mint leaves, washed, dried and roughly chopped
3 tablespoons water
pinch of salt (omit for babies)

In a food processor or blender, purée all the ingredients until smooth. Serve immediately.

Store in a sealed container in the refrigerator for up to 3 days.

> **For younger babies 7 months plus** who are into finger food, use this as a dipping sauce.
>
> **For older babies** serve as a dipping sauce with toast 'soldiers' (finger-sized pieces).
>
> **For toddlers** serve as for adults.

GREEN GODDESS CREAMY HERB DRESSING

MAKES 400 G (14 OZ)

PREP TIME: 5 MINUTES

This is a creamy, delicious sauce packed with leafy herbs. The gentle acid of the lemon plays beautifully against the combination of sweet tarragon, parsley and chives. It makes a simple cos (romaine) lettuce salad outrageously good.

250 g (9 oz/1 cup) mayonnaise
125 g (4½ oz/½ cup) sour cream
juice of ¼ lemon
1 garlic clove, finely crushed (just a tiny
    amount for babies)
1 very large handful of herbs, leaves
    only, such as flat-leaf/Italian parsley,
    chives and tarragon with perhaps a
    little sage, finely chopped
sea salt (omit for babies)
freshly ground black pepper (just a tiny
    amount for babies)

Whisk the mayonnaise and sour cream together until smooth. Add the lemon juice and whisk to combine. Add the garlic and all the chopped herbs, then season with salt and pepper to taste.

Store in a sealed container in the refrigerator for up to 3 days.

> **For younger babies 7 months plus and older babies**, before puréeing dilute with water or milk, as this is a creamy and rich dressing, and use as a dipping sauce or dressing for those who are into finger food.
>
> **For toddlers** serve as for adults.

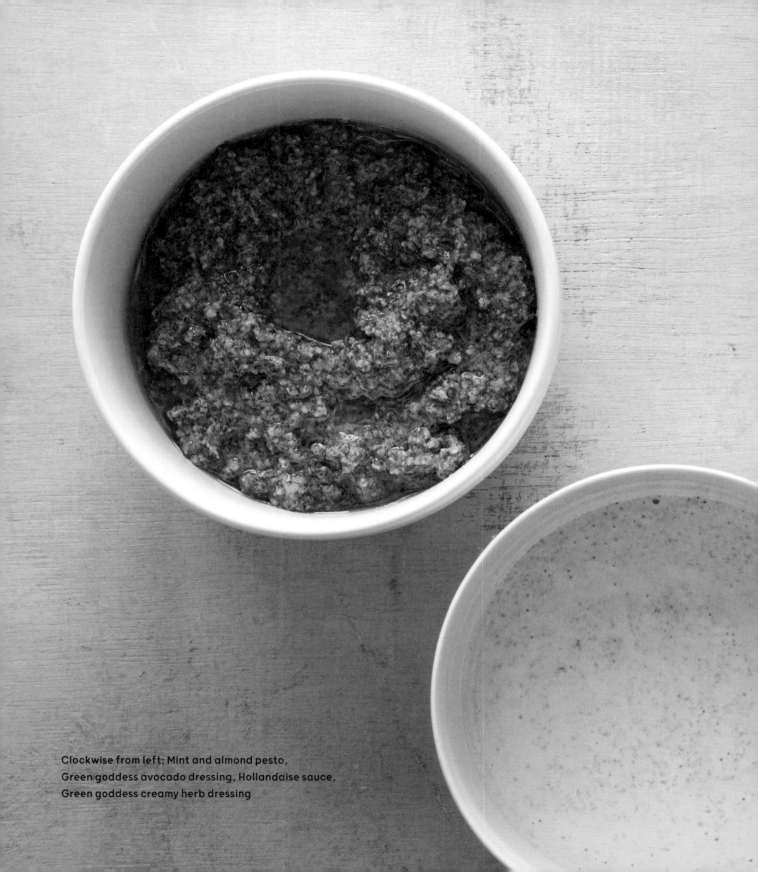

Clockwise from left: Mint and almond pesto,
Green goddess avocado dressing, Hollandaise sauce,
Green goddess creamy herb dressing

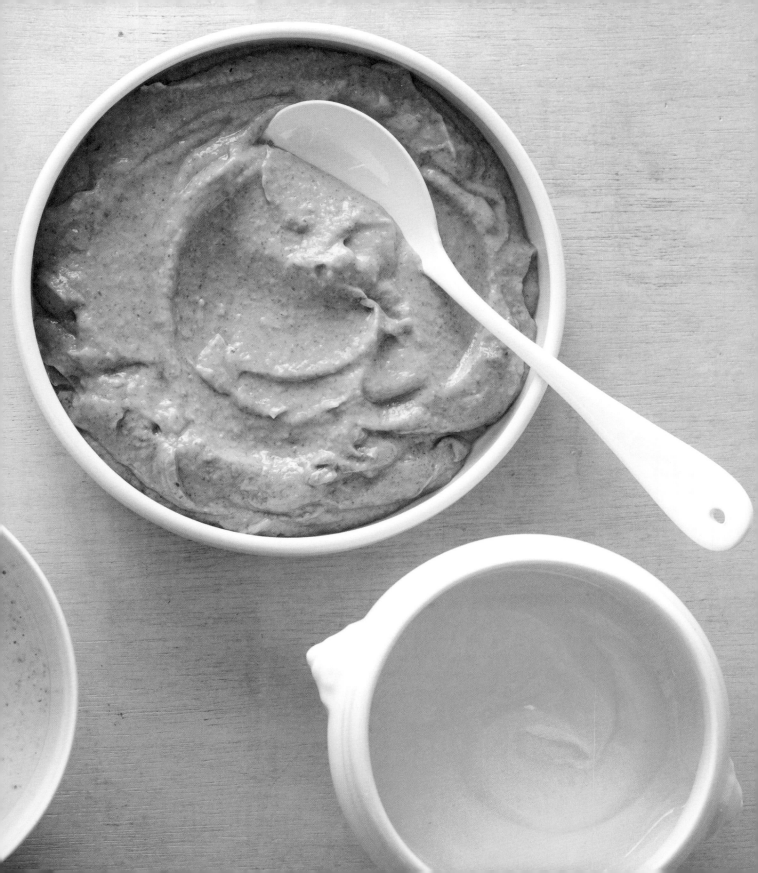

HOLLANDAISE SAUCE

Hollandaise is so easy to make at home – don't be scared, and remember practice makes perfect. It's so delicious and the perfect accompaniment for fish, seafood and steamed asparagus. Save the egg whites and freeze them to make meringues another time.

NOT FOR BABIES UNDER 12 MONTHS, AS EGG YOLKS MAY STILL BE RAW

MAKES 150 G (5¼ OZ/1 CUP)

PREP TIME: 10 MINUTES

COOKING TIME: 1 MINUTE

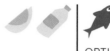

OPTIONAL

150 g (5¼ oz) butter
juice of ½ lemon
3 egg yolks
pinch of salt

Melt the butter slowly in a small saucepan over low heat.

Blend the lemon juice, egg yolks and salt in a food processor or blender until smooth and creamy, about 30 seconds. Gradually pour in the hot melted butter in a thin stream, with the food processor on medium speed. After all the butter is added, process for another 30 seconds to 1 minute.

If the sauce is not thick enough, you can further thicken it in a small saucepan over low heat for 30 seconds, whisking constantly. This needs your attention, so don't walk away! Remove the saucepan from the heat and continue to whisk the sauce for another 30 seconds. Pour into a serving bowl or storage container.

Store in the refrigerator for up to 2 days.

> **For toddlers** this is a delicious citrusy sauce to develop the flavour palate. Limit servings to just a couple of teaspoons, as it's rich.

ALMOND AÏOLI

NOT FOR BABIES UNDER 12 MONTHS DUE TO RAW EGG YOLKS

MAKES 550 G (1 LB 3 OZ/2 CUPS)

PREP TIME: 15 MINUTES

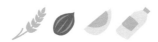

Aïoli can be made a few days ahead and stored in the refrigerator. The bread and almonds make this a more delicately flavoured aïoli than traditional versions.

1 slice ciabatta, crusts removed, roughly torn
100 ml (3½ fl oz) milk
250 ml (8½ fl oz/1 cup) grapeseed oil
250 ml (8½ fl oz/1 cup) extra virgin olive oil
2 egg yolks
2 garlic cloves, crushed
1 tablespoon lemon juice, plus extra as required
50 g (1¾ oz) finely ground almonds (see Note)
sea salt
ground white pepper

Put the torn bread into a small bowl and pour in the milk. Soak for 10 minutes, then squeeze the milk out of the bread and set aside.

Mix the grapeseed and olive oils together in a jug.

Add the egg yolks, garlic and lemon juice to a food processor and blend on high speed for 30 seconds to 1 minute until smooth. With the processor on low speed, slowly but steadily add the oils in a thin stream, then process until smooth and thick.

If the mixture is too thick, add a tablespoon of boiling water - this will relax the aïoli a little in texture and add shine to the sauce.

Add the ground almonds and soaked bread and blend thoroughly. Season to taste with salt and pepper and add a little extra lemon juice as required.

Cover and store in the refrigerator for up to 3 days - though this sauce is definitely best served at room temperature.

> **For toddlers** this is a great introduction to complex flavours as a dipping sauce. Limit the serving size, as it's rich.

NOTE: To make your own ground almonds, buy raw almonds (skin on) and grind them finely by blitzing them in a food processor.

ALMOND, GINGER AND COCONUT SAUCE

MAKES ABOUT 400 G (14 OZ/ 1¼ CUPS)

PREP TIME: 5 MINUTES

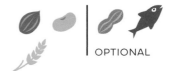

OPTIONAL

This is a fresh and healthy condiment. Enjoy it with steamed fish or roast chicken over a bowl of steamed rice with half an avocado on the side, or as an accompaniment to San choi bao with quinoa, peanuts and chicken (page 147) or a stir-fry.

250 ml (8¼ fl oz/1 cup) coconut milk
80 g (2¾ oz/½ cup) almonds
juice of 1 lime
2 tablespoons roughly chopped ginger
1 tablespoon soy sauce or gluten-free tamari (omit for babies)
1 teaspoon roughly chopped long red chilli (omit for babies)

Simply process all the ingredients together in a blender or food processor until smooth. If making for adults, check the sauce for the balance of lime (sour), soy (salty) and chilli (hot).

Store in a sealed container in the refrigerator for up to 3 days.

> **For younger babies** leave out the soy sauce and chilli.
>
> **For older babies** leave out the soy sauce and chilli. Serve with finely chopped fish or chicken and rice.
>
> **For toddlers** serve as for adults, but keep the chilli level low until they are ready for spicy foods at an older age.

PEANUT SAUCE

YIELDS ABOUT 400 G (14 OZ/ 1¼ CUPS)

PREP TIME: 5 MINUTES

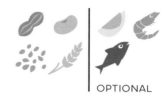

OPTIONAL

This is a robust Indonesian sauce. It's perfect served with thick-cut raw vegetables and hard-boiled egg, gado gado style. It also goes well with barbecued prawns (shrimp), steak, grilled white fish or chicken, beef or lamb skewers, meatballs or steamed rice, or you can finish a stir-fry with a spoonful. It can be spiced up for adults and older children with a love of spicy food, or toned down for toddlers and babies – see the variation.

250 g (9 oz/1 cup) smooth, unsalted peanut butter (see Home-made nut butters on page 217)

1 garlic clove, crushed

2 tablespoons lime juice

3 tablespoons hoisin sauce

½ teaspoon sesame oil

1 long red chilli, deseeded (use less if preferred)

2 tablespoons soy sauce

Add the peanut butter, garlic, lime juice, hoisin sauce, sesame oil and 125 ml (4 fl oz / ½ cup) water to a food processor and blitz to a smooth paste. At this point you can divide the batch into two - adults and kidlets. For adults and older children who like spice, add the chilli and soy sauce and blitz until smooth. Season to taste.

Store in a container in the refrigerator for up to 3 days.

> **For toddlers** who are more adventurous eaters, serve as for adults but omit or reduce the chilli.

Variation

1 tablespoon smooth, unsalted peanut butter (see Home-made nut butters on page 217)

3 tablespoons coconut cream

PEANUT SAUCE FOR BABY

To make a delicious simple peanut sauce for babies, process all the ingredients in a blender or food processor. Store in a sealed container in the refrigerator for up to 3 days.

> **For younger babies, older babies and toddlers** this baby-friendly sauce is a great way to introduce peanuts to meals.

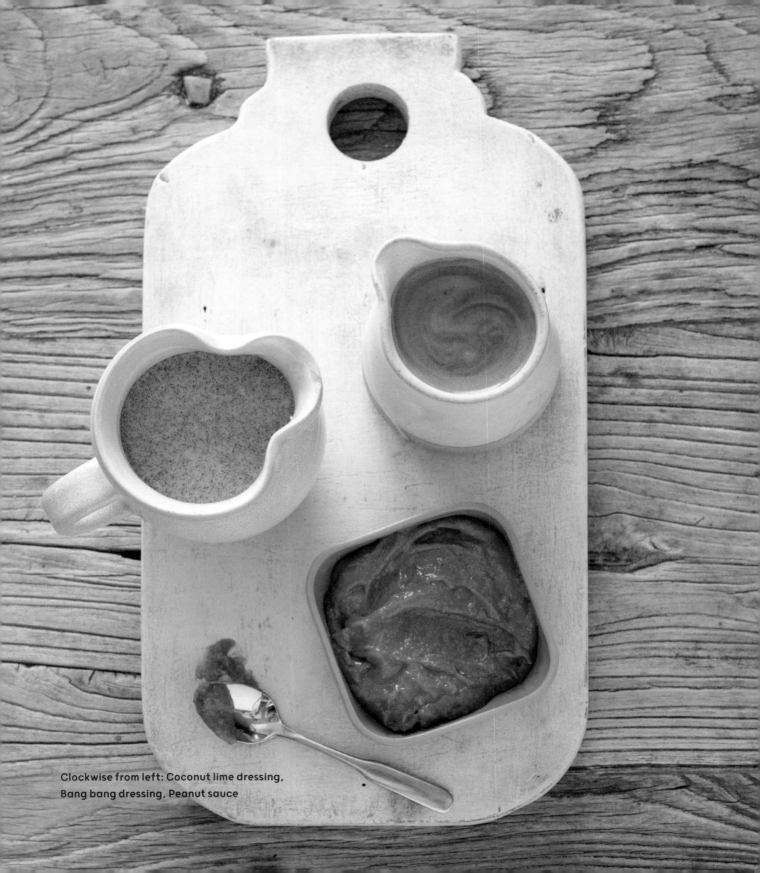

Clockwise from left: Coconut lime dressing,
Bang bang dressing, Peanut sauce

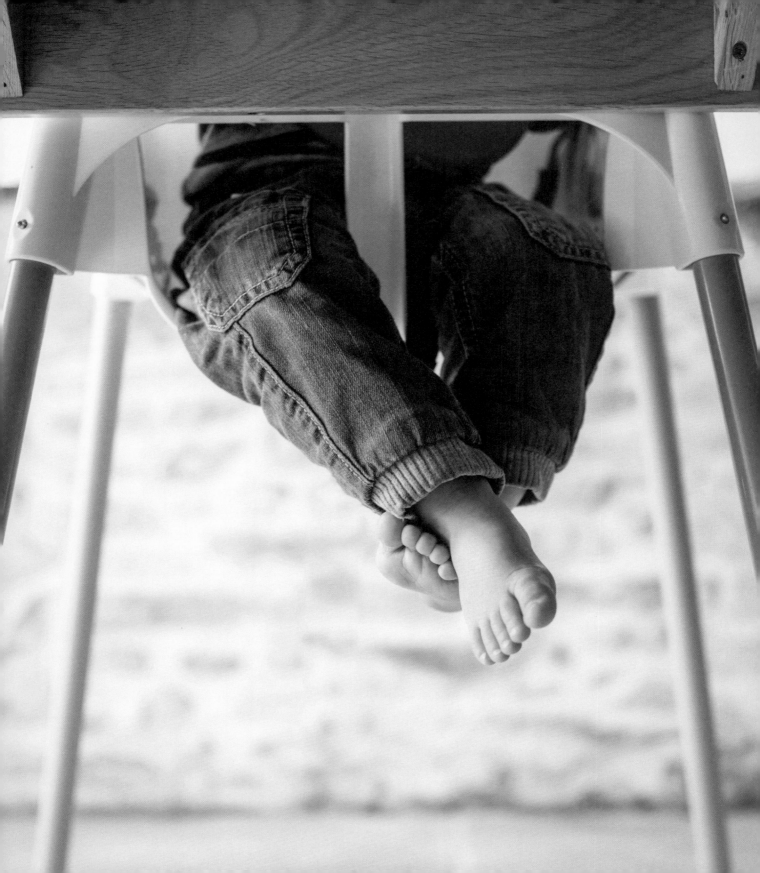

COCONUT LIME DRESSING

NOT SUITABLE FOR BABIES, AS IT'S TOO SALTY AND SPICY

MAKES ABOUT 400 G (14 OZ/1¾ CUPS)

PREP TIME: 5 MINUTES

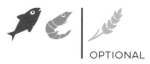

OPTIONAL

Perfect served with crisp apple or celery, fish fingers, chicken skewers or whole prawns (shrimp), and also wonderful as a dressing with a poached chicken and noodle salad, and as a dipping sauce for Rice paper rolls (page 149). This is a recipe for adults and children with a love of spicy food.

1 coriander (cilantro) root, well washed and roughly chopped
2 garlic cloves
1 long red chilli, deseeded
1 teaspoon brown sugar
juice of 1 lime
1 tablespoon fish sauce
250 ml (8½ fl oz/1 cup) coconut milk
pinch of salt

Add the coriander, garlic and chilli to a food processor and blitz to a fine paste. Add the sugar, lime juice, fish sauce and coconut milk and blitz again. Add salt to taste.

Store in a sealed container in the refrigerator for up to 3 days.

> **For toddlers** serve this to adventurous eaters, but watch the spice level for younger toddlers.

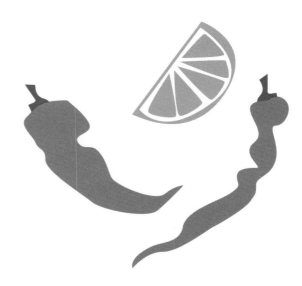

BANG BANG DRESSING

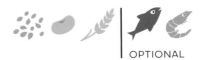

OPTIONAL

This is one of the great Asian sauces. It's creamy and a little bit sweet, and perfect in a classic chicken noodle salad. We love to use it as a dipping sauce with raw vegetables or barbecued meats and seafood. This is a treat for adults and children who love spicy food.

200 ml (7 fl oz) soy sauce or gluten-free
     tamari (omit for babies)
200 ml (7 fl oz) Chinese black vinegar
200 g (7 oz) white tahini
150 g (5¼ oz/1 lightly packed cup)
     coconut sugar
2 teaspoons sesame oil
1 teaspoon chilli oil
sea salt
ground white pepper

Blitz all the ingredients in a food processor until smooth - a hand-held blender also works well. Season to taste.

Store in a sealed container in the refrigerator for up to 3 days.

> **For toddlers** serve this to adventurous eaters, but watch the spice level for younger toddlers.

APPLE BUTTER WITH HAZELNUT, PRUNE AND CINNAMON

MAKES 785 G (1 LB 12 OZ/ 2½ CUPS)

PREP TIME: 10 MINUTES

COOKING TIME: 7 MINUTES

 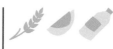

OPTIONAL

This is such a delicious fruit butter you'll want to eat it straight from the jar. Don't peel the apples – keep that superb colour that comes from the skins. If you want to swap the nuts, stay with sweet tree nuts such as almonds, cashew nuts or macadamia nuts. However, the nuts are optional. Serve with Classic porridge (page 66), Pikelets (page 85), pancakes or French toast (page 82) for breakfast, or at the end of the day with roast pork or other meats.

4 red apples, washed, cored and cut into small pieces
8 prunes, pitted and finely chopped
250 ml (8½ fl oz/1 cup) water
1 teaspoon hazelnut meal (easily made by finely grinding hazelnuts with skin on, or other nuts of choice, in a food processor)
pinch of ground cinnamon (just a tiny amount for babies)

Place all the ingredients, except the hazelnut meal, in a small saucepan. Bring to the boil over high heat, then reduce the heat and simmer for 5 minutes. Allow to cool, then purée with the hazelnut meal until smooth.

To store, pour into hot sterilised jars and seal when cold. This will keep in the refrigerator for up to 10 days.

> **For younger babies** this is great served with Baby's first cereal (page 58) or stirred through yoghurt.
>
> **For older babies** serve with porridge, pikelets or French toast.
>
> **For toddlers** serve as for adults.

HOME-MADE NUT BUTTERS

MAKES 250 G (9 OZ/1 CUP)

PREP TIME: 3-10 MINUTES

COOKING TIME: 8-12 MINUTES
IF ROASTING

OPTIONAL

Nut butters (pastes) are quick and easy to make at home – you just need a powerful food processor. You can make nut butters from raw or roasted nuts – raw nuts have a milder flavour than roasted nuts, which make a richer-tasting butter. Use nuts with the skins on for a fuller flavour. Have fun and experiment with nut combinations. We love to add extras to the blender, such as coconut butter, chia seeds, linseeds (flax seeds) or hemp seeds. Add in a few dates for sweetness, if desired.

1 cup raw nuts of your choice
2 teaspoons nut oil or other neutral-flavoured oil

If you are roasting the nuts first, preheat the oven to 180°C (350°F). Spread the nuts on a baking tray and roast for 8-12 minutes. Allow to cool.

Blend the nuts in a high-speed food processor for up to 10 minutes (see Note). The texture can be smooth or crunchy. Add just enough oil to get the nuts to a paste if the mixture is too dry.

To store, pour into hot sterilised jars and seal when cool. Store in the refrigerator for several weeks.

> **For younger babies** purée until smooth and serve with Baby's first cereal (page 58), or stir through yoghurt.
>
> **For older babies** you can make the purée slightly coarser, but ensure the nut pieces are fine crumbs.
>
> **For toddlers** serve as for adults.

NOTE: Nuts with a higher oil content, such as macadamia nuts and peanuts, make a paste in just a few minutes, whereas less oily nuts, such as almonds, hazelnuts and pecans, may require a much longer blending time.

HOME-MADE RICOTTA

MAKES 400 G (14 OZ/2 CUPS)

PREP TIME: 15 MINUTES

COOKING TIME: 15 MINUTES

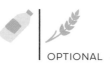

OPTIONAL

The joy of making ricotta from scratch far outweighs the chore! Ricotta is delicious sprinkled over salads, pasta, desserts and on toast at breakfast. For babies, it's a great substitute for sharper cheeses such as parmesan.

2 litres (68 fl oz/8 cups) full-cream
   (whole) cow's or goat's milk (see Note)
1 teaspoon sea salt
3 tablespoons freshly squeezed and
   strained lemon juice

Pour the milk into a large deep saucepan and place over medium heat, stirring occasionally with a wooden spoon. Add the sea salt and stir until dissolved. As the milk comes to the boil, lots of small bubbles will appear on the surface. At this point, stir the milk, then remove the spoon and pour in the lemon juice. Small lumps should start to rise to the surface as the milk curdles. The results with lemon juice can vary since it depends on the acidity of the lemon - add an additional tablespoon or two of lemon juice if your milk does not curdle immediately. Use the spoon to gently draw the curds into the centre of the pan to make room for more curds to rise at the edges.

Once the mixture starts to boil, remove the pan from the heat, cover, and leave for 15 minutes. Meanwhile, place 2 or 3 layers of muslin (cheesecloth) in a large strainer or sieve set over a large bowl.

Remove the lid from the pan and allow the steam to escape. Using a slotted spoon, gently lift the curds out of the pan, shaking the spoon to remove any excess liquid. Place the curds into the strainer. Alternatively, pour the mixture through the strainer, gently stirring to push all the liquid through.

Allow the curds to sit in the strainer for 15 minutes. Wrap the muslin around the curds and squeeze gently to remove more liquid. Allow to drain until the ricotta reaches a firm consistency. Don't over-squeeze or your ricotta will be too dense. Store, covered, in the refrigerator for up to 2 days.

NOTE: Very fresh milk (organic is always best) will easily separate into curds and whey.

For younger babies mix the ricotta through purées.

For older babies ricotta makes great finger food served on gnocchi and pasta or with mashed fruits.

For toddlers serve as for adults.

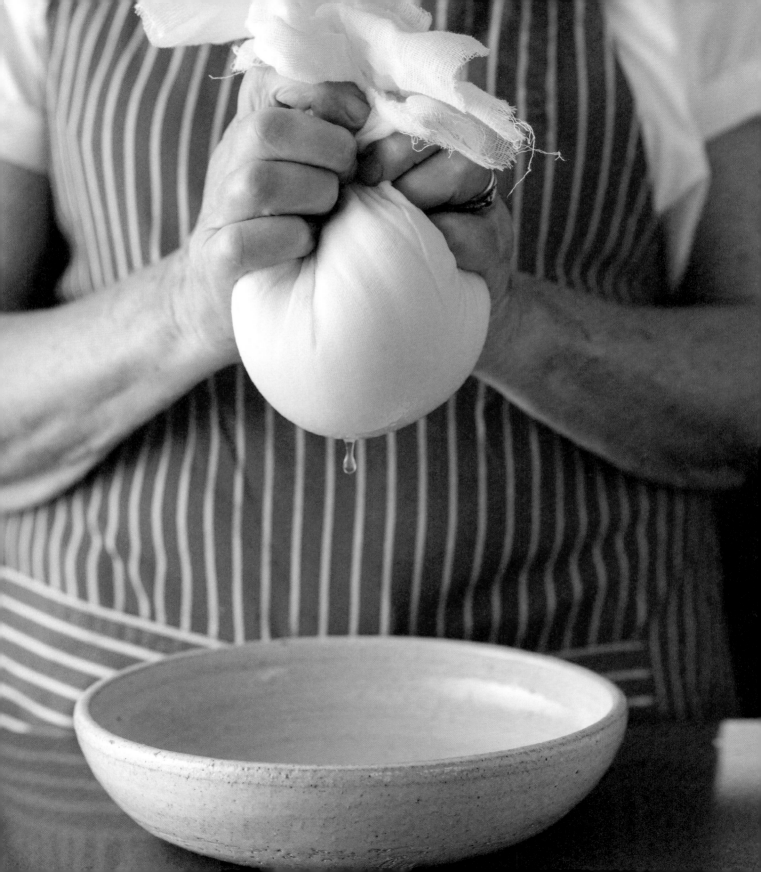

TASTY TOASTED SPRINKLE

MAKES 295 G (10¼ OZ/2¼ CUPS)

PREP TIME: 5 MINUTES

COOKING TIME: 5 MINUTES

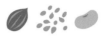

OPTIONAL

A savoury blend perfect to scatter on salads, meats or vegies, or to eat as a snack, this sprinkle can be served hot or cold. Feel free to substitute your favourite nuts for the almonds or mix it up with pistachio nuts and macadamia nuts.

80 g (2¾ oz/½ cup) finely chopped raw almonds, skin on

70 g (2½ oz/½ cup) pepitas (pumpkin seeds) 60 g (2 oz/½ cup) sunflower seeds

40 g (1½ oz/¼ cup) sesame seeds

2 teaspoons tamari (omit for babies)

Heat a heavy-based frying pan over high heat. When the pan is hot, add the almonds and seeds. Stir from time to time with a wooden spoon. When the nuts and seeds are starting to colour evenly, remove the pan from the heat and add the tamari. Keep stirring until the nuts and seeds are well coated and most of the moisture has been absorbed. Serve hot or leave to cool.

Store in an airtight container in the refrigerator for up to 5 days.

> **For younger babies** leave out the tamari and blitz the sprinkle to a fine powder in a blender or food processor. Stir sparingly into purées to add flavour.
>
> **For older babies** make sure the nuts are very finely chopped to avoid a choking risk.
>
> **For toddlers** serve as for adults.

POWERNUT CRUMBLE

MAKES ABOUT 755 G
(1 LB 11 OZ/3 CUPS)

PREP TIME: 5 MINUTES

COOKING TIME: 15 MINUTES

OPTIONAL

Powernut crumble has just a touch of mellow sweetness and is an ideal topping for puddings, or at breakfast on bircher. Jam-packed with essential fatty acids and all the good fats, this is the perfect addition to stewed fruit, yoghurt and ice cream.

160 g (5¼ oz/1 cup) macadamia nuts
80 g (2¾ oz/½ cup) raw almonds
40 g (1½ oz/¼ cup) peanuts (optional)
70 g (2¼ oz/½ cup) pepitas (pumpkin seeds)
3 tablespoons coconut oil, melted
135 g (5 oz/1½ cups) desiccated coconut
2 tablespoons maple syrup
1 teaspoon natural vanilla extract
pinch of ground cinnamon (just a tiny amount for babies)

Preheat the oven to 170°C (340°F). Line a baking tray with baking paper.

Blitz the nuts and pepitas in a food processor until coarse. Transfer to a mixing bowl and add the coconut oil, desiccated coconut, maple syrup, vanilla and cinnamon.

Spread on the baking tray and bake for 15 minutes. Allow to cool thoroughly, then transfer to an airtight container.

Store in the refrigerator for up to 5 days.

> **For younger babies** blitz the crumble to a fine powder in a blender or food processor and stir sparingly through yoghurt and bircher for breakfast.
>
> **For older babies** make sure the nuts are very finely chopped to avoid choking hazards.
>
> **For toddlers** serve as for adults.

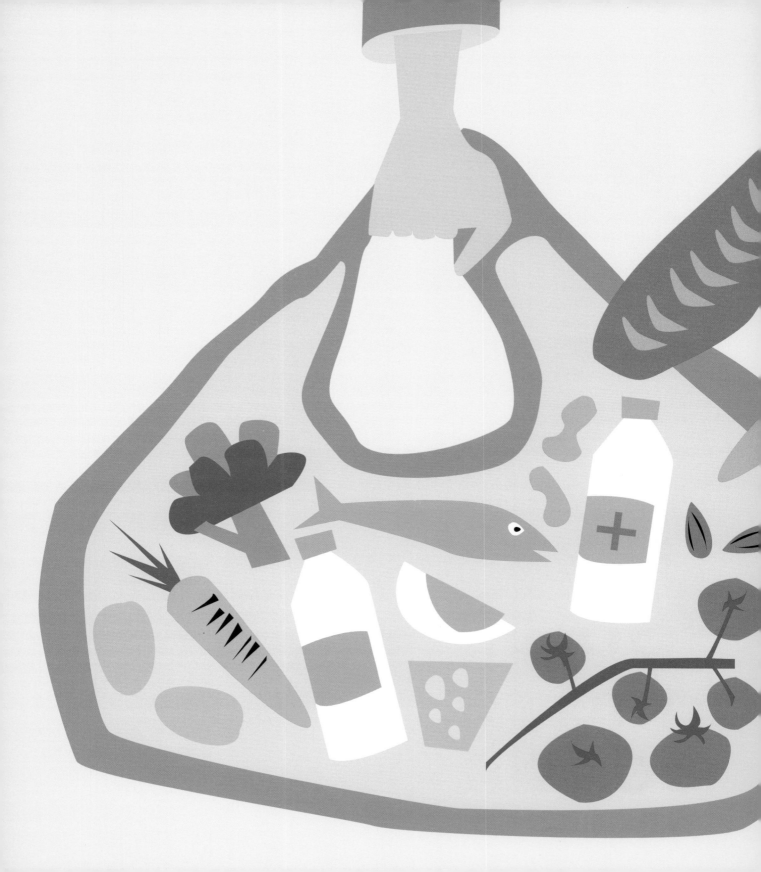

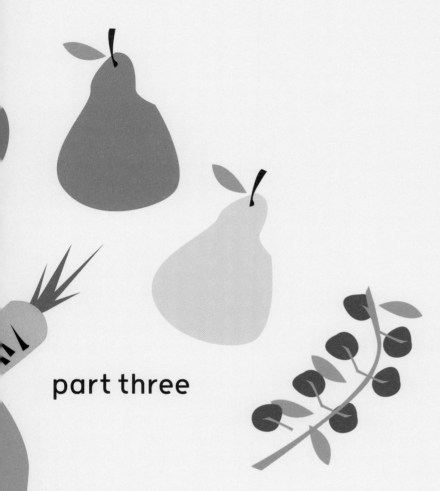

part three

Understanding food allergies and related conditions

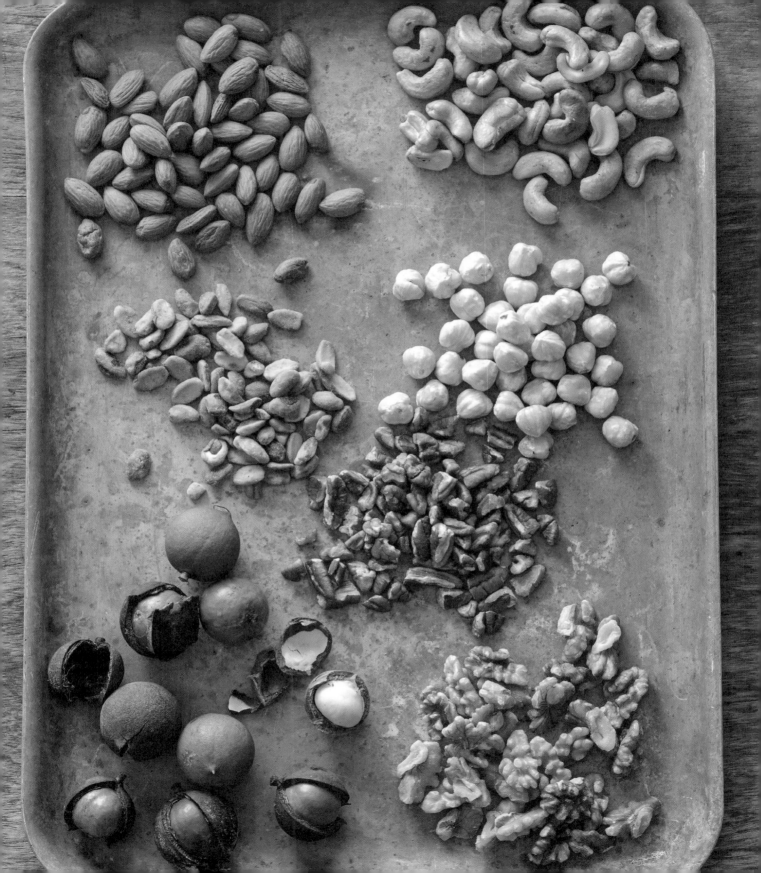

What are food allergies?

A food allergy is an overreaction of a child's (or adult's) immune system to a food protein. In an allergic reaction to a food, the immune system treats what is normally a harmless substance as a major threat and sets off the body's defences. The most common food allergens include peanuts, tree nuts, eggs, dairy, wheat, soy, sesame, fish and shellfish (see page 36), but this varies in different countries around the world. A food allergy can be diagnosed with skin-prick or blood tests. Allergy testing should only be carried out by a specialist allergist team.

An allergic reaction can vary from mild or moderate to severe. Symptoms range from skin redness, hives or welts, or swelling of the lips, eyes or face, to - in the most severe cases - vomiting, diarrhoea, difficulty breathing and anaphylactic shock. If you notice any of these symptoms, or any change in your baby's wellbeing (such as becoming very unsettled) soon after giving them a new food, they could be having an allergic reaction - stop feeding and seek medical advice.[9]

When a child has a severe food allergy, managing the allergy means avoiding all contact with the offending food or even traces of it.

SIGNS OF AN ALLERGIC REACTION

Contact your doctor if you notice signs of a mild to moderate reaction:

- **Swelling of the face or eyes**

- **Tingling in the mouth, swelling of the lips**

- **Hives or welts anywhere on the body**

- **Stomach pain and vomiting**

- **NOTE:** *A mild to moderate reaction can progress to anaphylaxis - even in those who have only ever had mild reactions before.*

Seek medical help immediately if you notice signs of a severe allergic reaction (anaphylaxis):

- **Difficult/noisy breathing**

- **Swelling of the tongue**

- **Swelling in the throat (e.g. drooling, difficulty swallowing)**

- **Change in voice or cry and/or difficulty vocalising**

- **Wheezing or persistent coughing**

- **Becoming pale and floppy (young children)**

- **Collapse**

SKIN SENSITIVITY VERSUS ALLERGIC REACTION

Skin sensitivity and the reddening of a child's skin on contact with some foods is not necessarily a diagnosis of a food allergy. Children, especially babies, have very sensitive skin and some foods that are higher in natural food chemicals, such as tomato, pineapple and strawberries, can irritate the skin. Gently wiping the skin clean with a moist cloth will in most cases allow any superficial irritation to settle. (See also Allergies and your baby's skin - dry skin and eczema on page 233.)

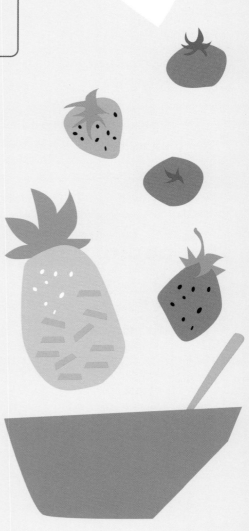

The immune system and food allergies

The immune system is your body's defence program. It is made up of specialised cells, organs, proteins and body tissue that work every day to defend the body against bacteria, viruses and microbes, which the body sees as foreign intruders. The immune system keeps the body healthy by fighting and preventing infections caused by these intruders. In a food allergy response, the body's immune system overreacts and treats what are normally harmless substances, such as certain foods, as a major threat and sets off the body's defences, causing various reactions (see Signs of an allergic reaction on page 225).

Some children are born with an overactive immune system, meaning their immune system may be more likely to become sensitive to some food allergens they come in contact with.[10] A child may have a family history of food allergies, in which case they are 60-80 per cent more likely to develop the food allergy. However, a small percentage of children without a family history may also go on to develop a food allergy. Some children with eczema or dry skin may be more susceptible - in their case, the food allergen contact is through dry, inflamed or broken skin (see page 233). However, being in the 'susceptible' category does not always mean a child will develop a food allergy.

Antibodies and mast cells

An antibody is a protein that is produced by the immune system. Immunoglobulin E (IgE) antibodies are produced by the immune system, which makes a specific IgE antibody to respond to specific allergens. Although everyone can make IgE antibodies, people who are prone to allergic reactions make much larger quantities.

Your child's immune response to a food is triggered by IgE antibodies, which are attached to mast cells. These mast cells are found on the skin, in the airways, throat and lungs, and in the gut - in other words, in places where the body is most likely to come into contact with an allergen. These mast cells are the body's early warning system. But just like conventional alarm systems, they can be set off by the wrong triggers.

When your child is allergic to something, they have a lot more IgE antibodies on their skin and in their airways and gut, waiting to warn and defend them. It's because each type of IgE is specific to each type of

In a food allergy response, the body's immune system overreacts and treats what are normally harmless substances as a major threat

allergen that some people are only allergic to peanuts, while others, who have many more types of IgE antibodies, react to multiple allergens.

Sensitisation can happen when a susceptible child forms allergen-specific IgE antibodies because they have repeated contact with a specific food protein but don't eat it (see page 236). The child's immune system has been sensitised and can create an allergic response when the food is eaten at a later time.

What happens when an IgE detects an allergen?

When the IgE antibodies detect their specific food allergen, the mast cells trigger the immune system. They release a series of chemicals, the most well known being histamine, which can cause symptoms such as itching and inflammation of the skin, wheezing in the lungs and tissue swelling; it can also make blood pressure drop. Other chemicals are also released by the cells – some have similar effects to histamines and others tell the body to produce even more IgE antibodies.

This reaction usually causes symptoms in the nose, lungs, throat or on the skin, and symptoms can vary from mild to life threatening. Even a mild reaction can develop into a more severe reaction if the body continues to produce IgE antibodies and other chemicals, escalating the allergic symptoms. (See Signs of an allergic reaction on page 225.)

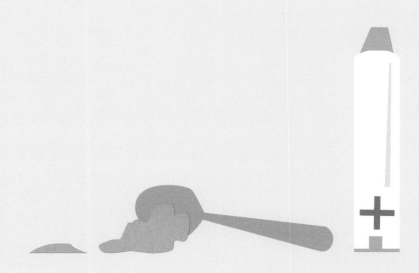

How we can reduce food allergies

Allergic diseases such as allergic asthma and hayfever have risen significantly around the world in the past 20 years, but are now seen to be more stable. As mentioned on page 8, while food allergies affect only about 4-8 per cent under the age of 5, today the fear for families is that the number of children developing food allergies has continued to rise concerningly, especially peanut and tree-nut allergies. And it's not just the children of people who already have allergies who are developing them, it's the children with no allergic history in their family.

Introduce food allergens early to avoid problems

In the past it was thought avoiding food allergens during pregnancy and childhood would prevent the development of food allergies. However, according to the research,[11] delaying the introduction of the common allergy-causing foods does not prevent food allergies.

Today the recommendations of many of the world's leading medical organisations of allergy experts, such as the British Society for Allergy and Clinical Immunology, the Australasian Society of Clinical Immunology and Allergy, and the American Academy of Allergy, Asthma and Immunology, now advise that introducing the common food allergens to your baby between the ages of 6 and 12 months may reduce the chance of your child developing a food allergy.[12] Once successfully introduced, and once your child has tolerance for each of these foods, you should continue to make them part of your child's diet on a regular basis.

It's easy to ignore food allergens and exclude them from your baby's meals without even realising it. Most of the processed and packaged children's foods are 'free from' and contain no food allergens. If your child is in a nut-free day care from the age of 4 months - which isn't uncommon these days for many working families - you only have the evening meal and weekends to introduce those foods to your child. **If you don't think of it consciously, it's easy for the first 12 months of your child's life to pass by without you introducing the common food allergens. It's important to introduce these foods deliberately at mealtimes or in snacks.** By introducing these foods before 12 months, your child will also experience a wider range of foods with a richer variety of flavours. (See Part One for more information on the common food allergens and introducing them to your baby's diet.)

A small percentage of babies may still go on to develop food allergies, despite you following the advice of experts that we have set out for you in this book.

Babies in the high-risk category

If your family has a history of food allergies or your child has dry skin or eczema, they are more vulnerable to developing food allergies. If a parent has a food allergy, their child has a 60-80 per cent chance of developing food allergies. You should then seek the advice of your doctor or paediatric allergist before introducing common food allergens.

If your child already has a diagnosed allergy, then you should avoid the food they are allergic to and substitute other foods. If they have extensive allergies, you may want to seek advice from a specialist dietitian to ensure you are providing a balanced diet and adequate nutrition while avoiding the food allergens.

If another member of the family has a food allergy, you should not necessarily avoid giving that food to your non-allergic child, but you should follow your doctor's advice. It's important to keep the family member with the food allergy safe, and to avoid cross-contamination during food preparation or any spoon sharing.

Growing out of allergies

Fortunately, nearly two-thirds of children with food allergies outgrow them by 4-6 years of age. The common food allergies that children are most likely to outgrow are egg, cow's milk, wheat and soy. Children are less likely to grow out of peanut and tree-nut allergies and, in fact, nut allergies are on the rise in Australia, the US and UK. Why do we outgrow food allergies? That is the question researchers are keen to solve. There are a few theories but no clear answers. Some experts believe that tolerance to some food allergens may develop as a child is exposed to very low levels of the allergen over time. We need more research to find the answers.

Other food allergens on the rise

We do know that allergies to some foods more commonly eaten in specific countries are on the rise. Buckwheat allergy, though rarely seen in Australia, the US and the UK, is seen as a common food allergen in Korea and Japan, where buckwheat is a daily staple. The frequency of buckwheat allergy is growing in Europe and other countries where buckwheat is being increasingly consumed, especially as part of a gluten-free diet.

Seafood and shrimp (prawns) are more common allergens in Asia, where they are often consumed daily and are also found in fish sauces used in cooking.

In Israel, where sesame has been a staple food for centuries, sesame allergy is becoming increasingly common - even more so than tree-nut or peanut allergies. The increased consumption of sesame in other countries has seen the sesame allergy rise around the world, as we use it daily in foods such as tahini, hummus, 'health' bars and other products.

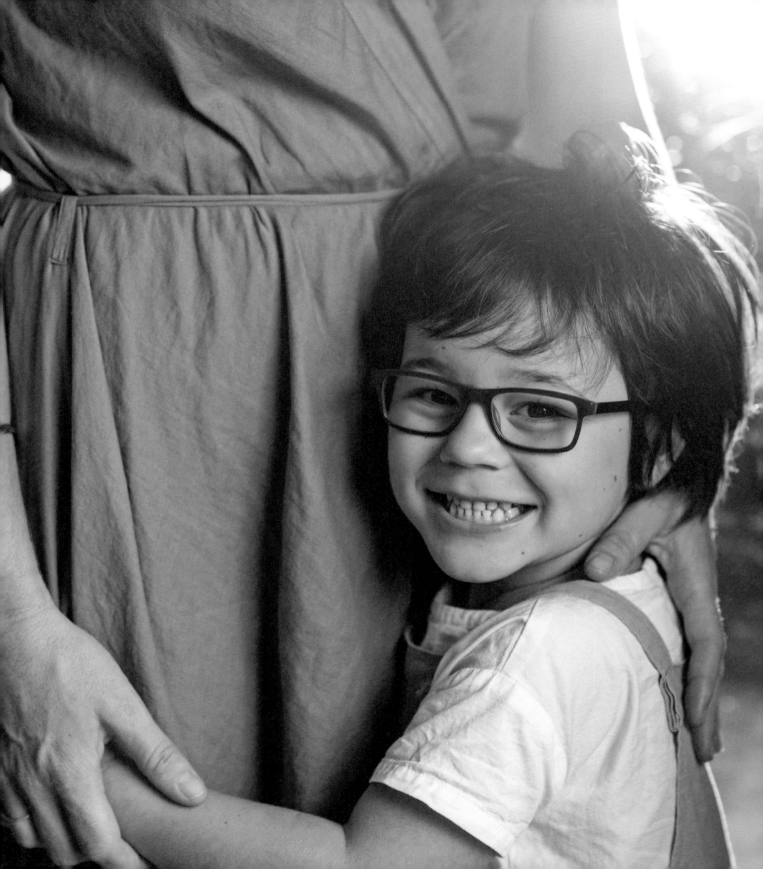

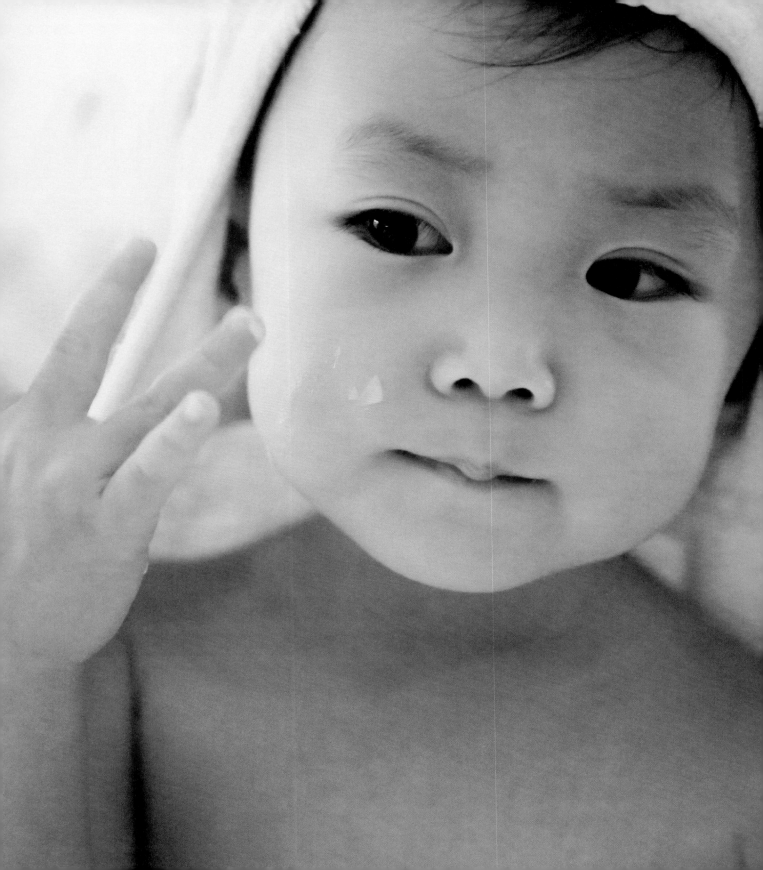

Allergies and your baby's skin – dry skin and eczema

The skin is the body's largest organ and its first line of defence against substances the body thinks are harmful. It acts as a barrier keeping bacteria and allergens out and keeping moisture in the body. Your child's skin plays a key role in allergy prevention and development. A baby's skin is more fragile and sensitive than an adult's skin. When the skin barrier is intact, your baby's skin should be plump and smooth.

Sensitisation to a food allergen can happen more easily when the skin surface is dry or microscopically broken. Instead of sitting on top of smooth, moist skin, the food proteins can more easily penetrate the skin and start an immune response. This is why children with dry skin or eczema are considered more susceptible to food allergies. Early treatment of dry skin or eczema in babies is important for your child's health and comfort.

Children with dry skin or eczema are also more likely to develop airborne allergens, asthma and hayfever. If there is a family history of food allergies or you are concerned about your child's dry skin or eczema, you should consult your doctor before introducing the common food allergens.

Dry skin

For babies, dry skin is rough or flaky to the touch but isn't red, itchy or inflamed. Dry skin can be general or can occur in patches, but is most commonly found on the face, arms and legs.

If your baby has dry skin, the skin barrier is weakened and not intact. Moisturising their skin helps maintain the skin barrier. (See Lotions, creams and oils on page 234.) There are excellent baby moisturisers that your doctor or pharmacist can recommend.

Eczema

Eczema is a condition where areas of your child's skin become inflamed, itchy, red, cracked and rough. It's sometimes called atopic dermatitis. In eczema the smooth barrier of the skin is disrupted and this allows food allergens to pass through more easily instead of repelling them. Therefore, treating and preventing eczema as much as possible in babies is very important.

The current recommendation is that the liberal use of moisturiser twice daily (even on days where there is no eczema) helps reduce skin dryness and form a moisture barrier over the skin. Parents can also help by preventing overheating and keeping children cool with cotton blankets and clothing, especially at night.

If your child's eczema doesn't improve within 48 hours of regular treatments, you should consult your doctor. Severe eczema should be managed in conjunction with your doctor.

Medical treatments for eczema may include:

- **Gentle skin moisturisers**
- **Diluted bleach baths for skin infections**
- **Antibiotics for severe skin infections**
- **Cortisone creams**
- **Moist body wraps and dressings**

Lotions, creams and oils

Face and hand creams for mum, and lotions and potions for baby, are among the most common new baby gifts. Some baby creams contain nut oils and dairy products, as do some hand creams, body washes and the like that the family may use. Do not use unrefined nut, dairy or sesame oils as moisturisers on your hands, face or on your baby. These oils can be readily absorbed through the skin and you can unknowingly sensitise your child to the food allergen in the cream.

It's been shown that the daily use of fragrance-free moisturising oils and creams that are also free from common allergens, for babies with dry skin, can help prevent the development of inflammations of the skin, such as eczema and dermatitis.[13]

Cleaning

Manufacturers today make disinfectants and cleaning products for every part of your house. We're told this is essential to keep your family safe, but not all microbes are bad. Researchers have shown that children develop fewer allergies when they grow up on farms or with a dog as a family pet.[14] The theory is that exposure to the many microbes found on a farm, or on the surface of your dog's coat, may enhance the early development of tolerance in your child's immune system.

Obviously, cleanliness and hygiene at home, proper cooking procedures and appropriate storage of food is important. Preventing cross-infection is a priority to make sure your child is protected from contagious diseases. COVID-19 awakened us to how important this is in the case of serious contagious diseases.

Washing your hands with soap and water is one of the best hygiene practices, as it prevents the spread of germs and infections. Teach your children to wash their hands before eating, after going to the toilet, and after touching anything that may be soiled or is likely to be contaminated with germs.

The sunshine vitamin

Vitamin D plays an important part in our immune system. Vitamin D is produced in the body through sunshine coming in contact with the skin. Studies in the US and Australia show that food allergies and eczema are much higher in the low sunshine areas furthest from the equator.[15] Vitamin D deficiency is associated with autoimmune diseases as well as an increased susceptibility to infection.

A healthy balance of exposure to sunshine and time outdoors is important for your child. However, avoid the hottest time of day or when the sun is strongest. Choose to spend short periods of time (5-10 minutes) in direct sunlight outdoors with your baby two to three times per week.

If you're spending prolonged periods outside, or you are outside during the time of day when the sun is intense, you need to protect your baby's delicate skin by moving them into the shade or covering them with protective clothing, or using a low-chemical, natural mineral sunscreen.

Vitamin D supplements for infants are not recommended. You can naturally increase the vitamin D in your child's diet with foods rich in this nutrient, such as oily fish including salmon, tuna and sardines. Other lower level sources of vitamin D include egg yolks, mushrooms, beef liver and cheese.

Sensitisation and developing oral tolerance

The common food allergens your child makes contact with are those they touch, feel and breathe in every day. **For most children this is not a problem – only for those with a genetic predisposition to allergy and eczema.** Microscopic traces of food proteins on the faces, fingertips, skin and clothes of loving parents, carers and friends can be transferred through kisses and cuddles. The protein may be present on the toys, floors, cutlery, benchtops, tables, phones, digital tablets, computer keyboards or the family car - everything that surrounds your baby and that their skin can make contact with.

If your child is in the susceptible category, take a close look at what's in your refrigerator and food cupboards, the snacks your family eats, and what you eat every day and the foods that surround your child. For example, if you eat peanuts regularly, the peanut protein will regularly be present in house dust on the benches and other surfaces of your home.

If you surround a susceptible baby with common food allergens but don't feed them to your child as part of their normal diet, their only allergen contact will be on their skin or in their environment – in such cases, the allergy risk dramatically increases and the susceptible child may become sensitised.

Becoming sensitised happens when a susceptible child forms allergen-specific IgE antibodies because they have repeated contact with a specific food protein but don't eat it. The child's immune system has then been sensitised and can create an allergic response when the food is eaten at a later time.

Developing oral tolerance

Oral tolerance to a food protein occurs when the gut creates specific tolerant antibodies to the food, or alternately no immune response happens at all.

A food allergy is seen as a breakdown in normal 'oral tolerance'. The food protein's regular contact with the child's skin triggers the immune system to create IgE antibodies in cells on the skin (see page 227). In susceptible children, oral tolerance may not develop if the child has repeated contact with the food allergen but does not eat it.

It's important to recognise that children who develop food allergies are still likely to be tolerant to most foods in their diets. Many are allergic to only one food, although some may be allergic to multiple foods (very rarely more than five).

Cautious introduction is always an important principle when introducing allergens to your baby. For more information see When and why to start introducing the common food allergens on page 34 and Babies in the high-risk category on page 230.

Coeliac disease, wheat allergy and wheat/gluten intolerance

Many families may be confused about the difference between food allergies and food intolerances, as well as wheat allergy, wheat and gluten intolerance and coeliac disease. Here are some brief explanations to help you understand the differences.

Food intolerances

A food intolerance is different from a food allergy and doesn't involve the immune system. Intolerances are reactions triggered by chemicals that are naturally found in food, such as salicylates, amines and glutamate, or by additives in food, such as MSG, artificial colours and flavours. These chemicals create a reaction that irritates the nerve endings in different parts of the body.

Typical food-intolerance symptoms in your baby can include:

- **Restlessness and irritability**
- **Inability to settle**
- **Colic**
- **Diarrhoea**
- **Eczema (see page 233)**
- **Recurring hives and rashes**
- **Behavioural problems in toddlers, such as attention deficit hyperactivity disorder (ADHD)**

A food intolerance can be quite challenging to diagnose and manage. It may be diagnosed by an elimination diet under the guidance of a specialist allergy team, to detect which food or foods are causing the problem. We haven't gone into detail on food intolerances in this book. However, there are some excellent resources written by medical experts on the area of childhood food intolerances and elimination diets.[16] If you think your child has a food intolerance you should consult your doctor or paediatric allergist before limiting your child's diet.

Coeliac disease

Coeliac disease is an autoimmune disease of the gut. Eating gluten triggers an abnormal reaction in the child's immune system, creating inflammation of the small intestine. This damages your child's ability to absorb healthy nutrients. Typical symptoms include diarrhoea, decreased appetite, stomach ache and bloating, poor growth and weight loss. Children with coeliac disease cannot eat any food that contains gluten.

Coeliac disease can only develop in children who are genetically susceptible. They carry genes called HLA-DQ2 or DQ8. About 30 per cent of the population can carry these genes, but coeliac disease only occurs in about 1 per cent of the population.[17] So even though parents or family members may have coeliac disease, that does not automatically mean that their children will develop it. Only a small percentage of those who are genetically at risk will develop the disease.

Early diagnosis is important to prevent damage to your child's health. Coeliac disease needs to be diagnosed by your doctor. Your child must be eating gluten/wheat when tested to get an accurate result, so do not remove it from their diet before the test. This is done through blood tests and, if these are positive, an endoscopy will be carried out. An endoscopy is done while your child is sedated or asleep, by a paediatric gastroenterologist, who will use a small, flexible camerascope to examine your child's small intestine and take a biopsy of the bowel lining. Many children with coeliac disease are diagnosed between 6 months and 2 years old, which is when most kids get their first taste of gluten in foods.

There has been much research done into the possible prevention of coeliac disease, but none of the results are conclusive. The age you introduce gluten to your child's diet, whether it's 4 months, 12 months or older, has not been found to make a difference to the development of coeliac disease in susceptible children. The treatment for coeliac disease is a lifelong gluten-free diet.

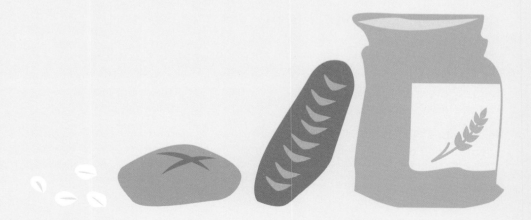

> ### GLUTEN-FREE DIET
>
> Diet has a major role to play in the development of a healthy gut for your child. If your child has coeliac disease or a diagnosed wheat or gluten intolerance, there is plenty of information and advice available from coeliac organisations. See our links in the Notes section.[18] Sound nutritional basics are still essential. The best start is to give your child a balanced diet of fresh food prepared at home - preferably organic.

Wheat allergy

Wheat allergy is very different from coeliac disease or gluten intolerance. While coeliac disease is an autoimmune reaction, wheat allergy is an immune reaction. Specifically, it is an immune overreaction to the protein in wheat, whereas coeliac disease is an autoimmune reaction to gluten.

Symptoms of a wheat allergy will be typical of an allergic reaction. If you notice any swelling of the lips, eyes or face, hives or welts, vomiting, or any change in your baby's wellbeing (such as becoming very unsettled) soon after eating food containing wheat, they could be having an allergic reaction. Stop feeding your baby that food and seek medical advice immediately.

Wheat and gluten intolerance

Gluten is a protein found mainly in wheat (and wheat varieties, such as spelt, kamut, durum, graham and semolina), barley, rye, triticale and malt (unless the malt comes from a non-wheat source).

Some children may develop an intolerance to gluten and other components in wheat, but this is not coeliac disease. The symptoms are mild and uncomfortable, and include bloating, abdominal pain, diarrhoea and constipation. Unlike in coeliac disease, the small bowel is not damaged and the child does not have problems absorbing nutrients from their food.

It's very important that before you remove wheat or gluten from your child's diet, you talk to your doctor, as there can be many other reasons for these symptoms. Researchers are not sure whether gluten or other compounds in wheat are always the problem in what appears to be a wheat or gluten intolerance.

Unless your child has a family history of wheat allergy or coeliac disease, you can introduce wheat to their diet as part of their regular meals from 6 months. Grains containing gluten are also rich in fibre, B vitamins, iron, magnesium and selenium, all essential for your baby's health. Children with a wheat allergy or intolerance - but not coeliac disease - can eat other grains such as oats, barley and rye.

Reflux

Why a section on reflux in a book about children's first foods and food allergies, you may ask. There are many medical conditions that may mimic reflux, including allergies, and this section is designed to explain some basics to help you understand the symptoms and presentation of reflux.

Babies and reflux

Reflux is one of the most unrecognised and underdiagnosed health issues in babies and toddlers.[19] Societal changes in diet and lifestyle have also contributed to a rise in reflux in both children and adults.

Very young babies have tiny tummies and a short oesophagus, so it's normal for them to spit up food. Babies need to burp - air bubbles accumulate in their tummies each time they swallow when breast or bottle feeding. Burping your baby lets them release the air, and a substantial baby 'burp' is often accompanied by a milky message all over the unsuspecting cuddler's clothes. It's normal for young babies to spit up food after feeding, and sometimes to vomit after a big feed when their tummies are overfull and the air has nowhere to go.

The reflux baby, however, is often the 'difficult' baby who is always uncomfortable and can't settle. Having a baby with reflux can truly test the fabric of a family. Hours of deprived sleep for parents, baby, and often the rest of the family, can put strain on relationships and wear everyone down. The reflux baby will often wake frequently in the night - every few hours - crying in pain. Daytime sleeps may be only 10-40 minutes, and baby will wake in distress. The reflux baby will be much more comfortable being cuddled in the fully upright position. When you lay them down, they may cry from genuine pain.

It's a fine line sometimes between what is considered normal and when you should seek your doctor's help. Regular projectile vomiting and vomiting during sleep is not considered healthy or normal for babies.

Reflux in babies and toddlers can also present silently in many other ways, with symptoms that go completely under the radar, including nasal congestion, noisy breathing, recurring cough or croup, or a constant runny nose. These symptoms may be easily misconstrued as allergies, coughs and colds. If in doubt seek your doctor's advice. Older children with reflux will have restless sleeping patterns and wake frequently.

Note that the recipes in Part Two of this book are not recipes to treat reflux. If you or your children have reflux, you should follow your doctor's or dietitian's recommendations. If you think your child has reflux you should consult your family doctor or paediatrician, who will examine your child thoroughly and give you the best advice.

What is acid reflux?

After food is swallowed it travels down the oesophagus to the stomach. At the entrance to the stomach there is a sphincter that opens and allows the food to enter, and then closes to keep the food inside, where your baby's stomach acids activate an enzyme called pepsin to digest the food. Acid reflux happens when the sphincter opens and allows recently eaten food and acidic stomach contents to go back up the oesophagus, which causes irritation and, in some cases, extreme discomfort.

What is respiratory reflux?

Respiratory reflux is when the acidic stomach contents and acidic foods flow back out of the stomach up to the mouth, nose and lungs. Respiratory reflux is acid reflux that causes ear, nose, throat and voice problems, and can cause serious lung problems, including asthma, coughs or chronic bronchitis.

FOOD CHOICES TO AVOID REFLUX

The basic guidelines below apply to families with diagnosed reflux. For specific foods and guidance you should follow your doctor's or dietitian's recommendations.

- **Avoid a diet rich in processed food, fast food, high-fat foods and sweet soft drinks.**

- **Fresh food cooked at home, including fruit and vegetables daily, is ideal. That means fresh, not tinned, food. Tinned, processed foods are made more acidic to preserve them.**

- **Keep serving sizes sensible.**

- **Make sure you and your children have time to digest your meals before bedtime, and avoid bedtime snacks.**

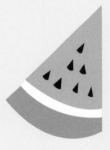
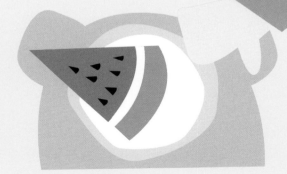

The need for more research

Researchers from around the globe have been looking into why food allergies are on the rise and how to prevent their development in children. They've looked at everything - the changing ways we eat, the increasing amount of processed food we eat, our environment, the amount of time our kids spend in the sunshine, and our obsession with cleanliness. Do they have all the answers? Not yet, but we are much better informed today, and new discoveries continue to move our knowledge forward.

The research around environmental exposure and the development of food allergies in children is still ongoing, and there is still much more work to be carried out on other factors that influence the development of childhood food allergies. The need for more research on the prevention and treatment of food allergies is essential. Research on this health issue is underfunded compared to many other areas of medicine. It is very important that governments and industry fund further research so that we can find solutions to the cause, management and treatment of food allergies.

> To make a difference to allergy research, please donate at www.slhd.nsw.gov.au/RPA/donation.html and direct your donation to the Velencia Soutter Memorial Fund.

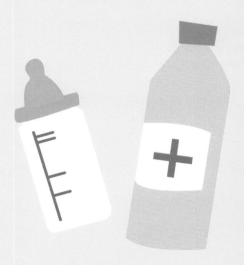

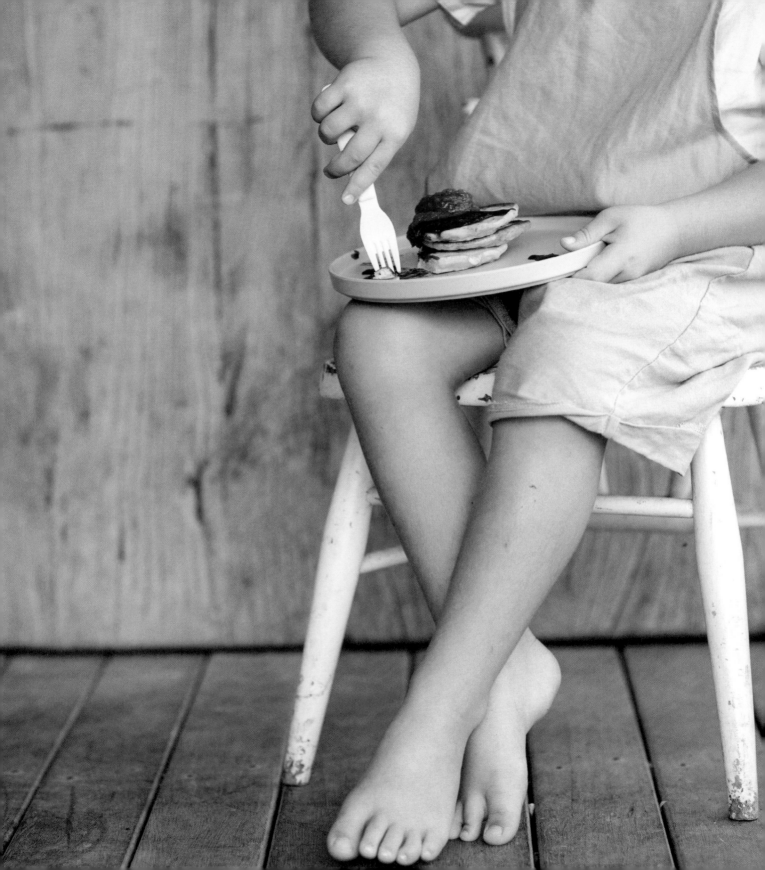

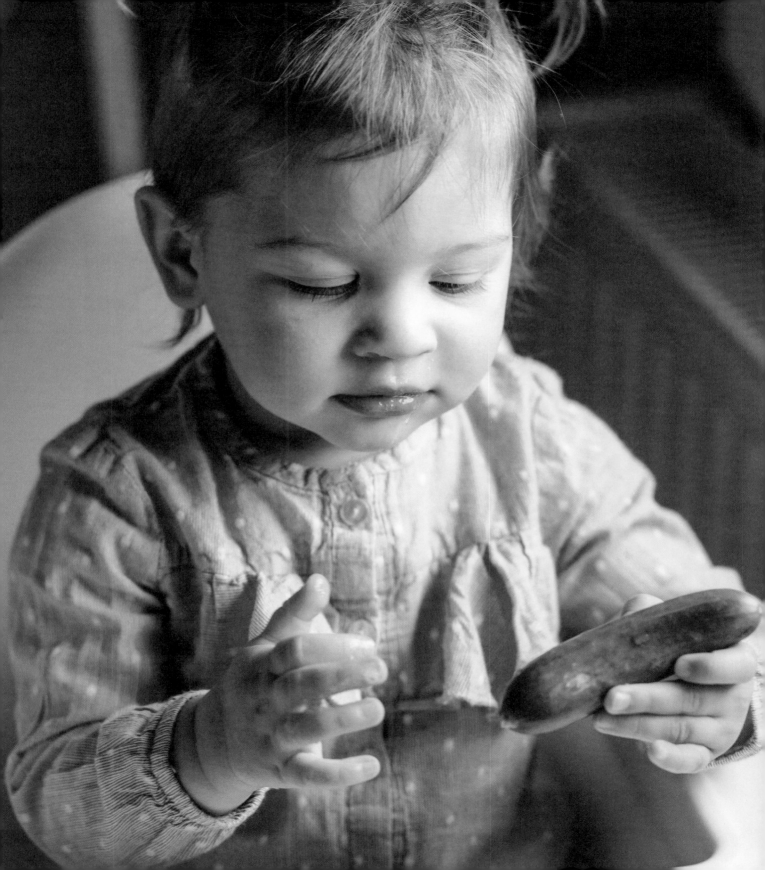

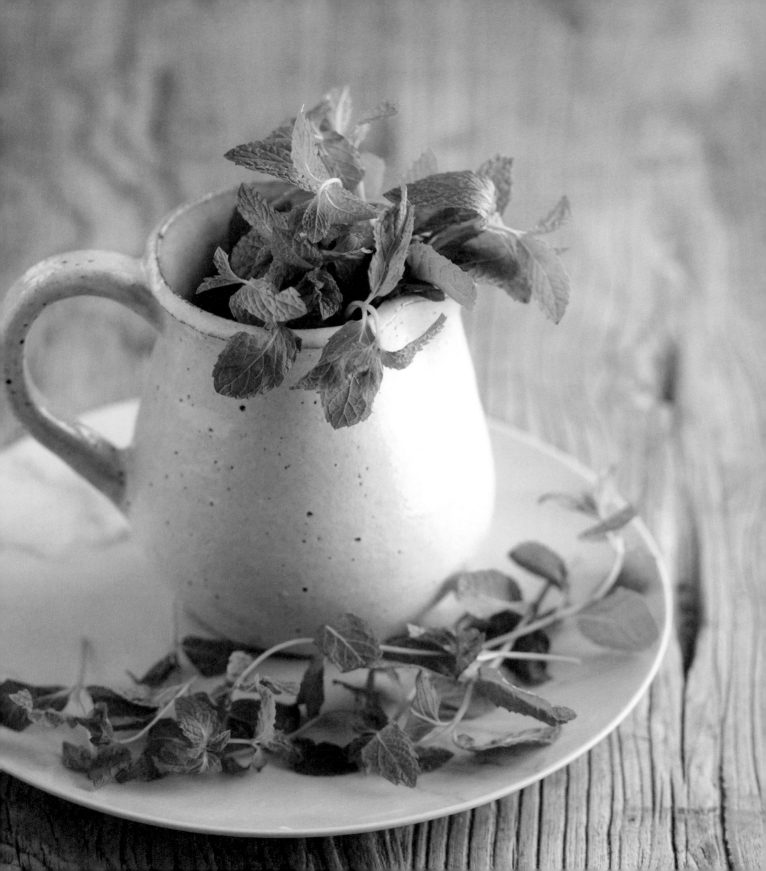

Notes

PART ONE

Home cooking creates healthier families

1. A. Swain, V. Soutter and R. Loblay, *Friendly Food: The Essential Guide to Managing Common Food Allergies and Intolerances*, new edition, Sydney, Murdoch Books, 2019

2. M.J. Harbec and L.S. Pagani, 'Associations between early family meal environment quality and later well-being in school-age children', *Journal of Developmental & Behavioral Pediatrics*, February/March 2018, Vol. 39, Issue 2, retrieved from www.pubmed.ncbi.nlm.nih.gov/29227338

When is my baby ready for solid food?

3. Dr J. Koufman, MD, FACS, Dr J. L. Wei, MD and Dr K.B. Zur, MD et al., *Acid Reflux in Children: How Healthy Eating Can Fix Your Child's Asthma, Allergies, Obesity, Nasal Congestion, Cough and Croup*, Simon & Schuster, 2018

4. More information on baby-led weaning can be found at:

    Cleveland Clinic: www.health.clevelandclinic.org/ 8-tips-for-introducing-solid-foods-with-baby-led-weaning

    BabyCenter: www.babycenter.com.au/a1007100/ baby-led-weaning

5. For information on how to perform first aid for children who show signs of choking, see the useful links below:

    St John's Ambulance video: www.youtube.com/ watch?v=oswDpwzbAV8

    Australian parenting website: www.raisingchildren.net. au/babies/safety/choking-strangulation/choking-first-aid-pictures

When and why to start introducing the common food allergens

6. Australasian Society of Clinical Immunology and Allergy (ASCIA): www.allergy.org.au/images/pcc/ASCIA_ Guidelines_infant_feeding_and_allergy_prevention.pdf

    American Academy of Allergy, Asthma & Immunology: www.aaaai.org/conditions-and-treatments/library/ allergy-library/prevention-of-allergies-and-asthma-in-children

    The British Society for Allergy & Clinical Immunology: www.bsaci.org/wp-content/uploads/2020/02/ pdf_Infant-feeding-and-allergy-prevention-PARENTS-FINAL-booklet.pdf

Nutritional basics

7. M. Pollan, *The Omnivore's Dilemma: The Search for a Perfect Meal in a Fastfood World*, London, Bloomsbury, 2011

8. Newcastle University, 'Importance of infant diet in establishing a healthy gut', *Science Daily*, 24 October 2018, retrieved from www.sciencedaily.com/ releases/2018/10/181024131243.htm

PART THREE

What are food allergies?

9. Australasian Society of Clinical Immunology and Allergy (ASCIA): www.preventallergies.org.au/identifying-allergic-reactions/

    British Red Cross: www.redcross.org.uk/first-aid/learn-first-aid-for-babies-and-children/allergic-reaction

The immune system and food allergies

10. University of Rochester Medical Center: www.urmc.rochester.edu/encyclopedia/content.aspx?ContentID=123&ContentTypeID=134

How we can reduce food allergies

11. Australasian Society of Clinical Immunology and Allergy (ASCIA): www.allergy.org.au/images/pcc/ASCIA_Guidelines_infant_feeding_and_allergy_prevention.pdf

    ASCIA Guide for the introduction of peanut to infants with severe eczema and/or food allergy: www.allergy.org.au/images/stories/pospapers/ASCIA_HP_guide_introduction_peanut_infants_2017.pdf

    G. Du Toit, P.H. Sayre, G. Roberts et al., 'Effect of avoidance on peanut allergy after early peanut consumption', The New England Journal of Medicine, 14 April 2016, retrieved from www.nejm.org/doi/full/10.1056/NEJMoa1514209

    G. Du Toit, G. Roberts, P.H. Sayre et al., 'Randomized trial of peanut consumption in infants at risk for peanut allergy', The New England Journal of Medicine, 26 February 2015, retrieved from www.nejm.org/doi/full/10.1056/NEJMoa1414850

    D.M. Fleischer, S. Sicherer, M. Greenhawt et al., 'Consensus communication on early peanut introduction and the prevention of peanut allergy in high-risk infants', The Journal of Allergy and Clinical Immunology, August 2015, retrieved from www.ncbi.nlm.nih.gov/pubmed/26122934

    A.W. Gunaratne, M. Makrides and C.T. Collins, 'Maternal prenatal and/or postnatal n-3 long chain polyunsaturated fatty acids (LCPUFA) supplementation for preventing allergies in early childhood', The Cochrane Database of Systematic Reviews, 22 July 2015, retrieved from www.ncbi.nlm.nih.gov/m/pubmed/26197477/

    M.S. Kramer and R. Kakuma, 'Maternal dietary antigen avoidance during pregnancy or lactation, or both, for preventing or treating atopic disease in the child', The Cochrane Database of Systematic Reviews, 12 September 2012, retrieved from www.ncbi.nlm.nih.gov/pubmed/22972039

    C.J. Lodge, K.J. Allen, A.J. Lowe et al., 'Overview of evidence in prevention and aetiology of food allergy: a review of systematic reviews', International Journal of Environmental Research and Public Health, 4 November 2013, retrieved from www.ncbi.nlm.nih.gov/pubmed/24192789

    D.J. Palmer, J. Metcalfe, M. Makrides et al., 'Early regular egg exposure in infants with eczema: a randomized controlled trial', The Journal of Allergy and Clinical Immunology, August 2013, retrieved from www.jacionline.org/article/S0091-6749(13)00762-8/pdf

    M.R. Perkin, K. Logan, A. Tseng et al., 'Randomised trial of introduction of allergenic foods in breast-fed infants', The New England Journal of Medicine, 5 May 2016, retrieved from www.nejm.org/doi/full/10.1056/NEJMoa1514210

12. Australasian Society of Clinical Immunology and Allergy (ASCIA): www.preventallergies.org.au

    American Academy of Allergy, Asthma and Immunology: www.aaaai.org/conditions-and-treatments/library/allergy-library/prevention-of-allergies-and-asthma-in-children

    The British Society for Allergy & Clinical Immunology: www.bsaci.org/wp-content/uploads/2020/02/pdf_Infant-feeding-and-allergy-prevention-PARENTS-FINAL-booklet.pdf

Allergies and your baby's skin – dry skin and eczema

13. K. Horimukai, MD, K. Morita, MD and M. Narita, MD et al., 'Application of moisturizer to neonates prevents development of atopic dermatitis', *The Journal of Allergy and Clinical Immunology*, Vol. 34, Issue 4, 1 October 2014, retrieved from www.jacionline.org/article/S0091-6749(14)01160-9/fulltext

14. B. Hesselmar, A. Hicke-Roberts, A.C. Lundell et al., 'Pet-keeping in early life reduces the risk of allergy in a dose-dependent fashion', *PLOS ONE*, 19 December 2018, retrieved from www.journals.plos.org/plosone/article?id=10.1371/journal.pone.0208472

15. N.J. Osborne, PhD, O.C. Ukoumunne, PhD, M. Wake MBChB, FRACP, MD et al., 'Prevalence of eczema and food allergy is associated with latitude in Australia', *Journal of Allergy and Clinical Immunology*, Vol. 129, Issue 3, March 2012, retrieved from www.jacionline.org/article/S0091-6749(12)00031-0/fulltext

Coeliac disease, wheat allergy and wheat/gluten intolerance

16. A. Swain, V. Soutter and R. Loblay, *Friendly Food: The Essential Guide to Managing Common Food Allergies and Intolerances*, new edition, Sydney, Murdoch Books, 2019

17. C. Meijer, R. Shamir, H. Szajewska et al., 'Celiac disease prevention', *Frontiers in Pediatrics*, 30 November 2018, retrieved from www.frontiersin.org/articles/10.3389/fped.2018.00368/full

18. For more information on Coeliac disease, gluten testing and gluten-free diets see the following coeliac organisations' websites:

Coeliac Australia: www.coeliac.org.au

Coeliac UK: www.coeliac.org.uk

Celiac Disease Foundation (US): www.celiac.org

Reflux

19. Dr J. Koufman, MD, FACS, Dr J.L. Wei, MD, Dr K.B. Zur, MD et al., *Acid Reflux in Children: How Healthy Eating Can Fix Your Child's Asthma, Allergies, Obesity, Nasal Congestion, Cough and Croup*, Simon & Schuster, 2018

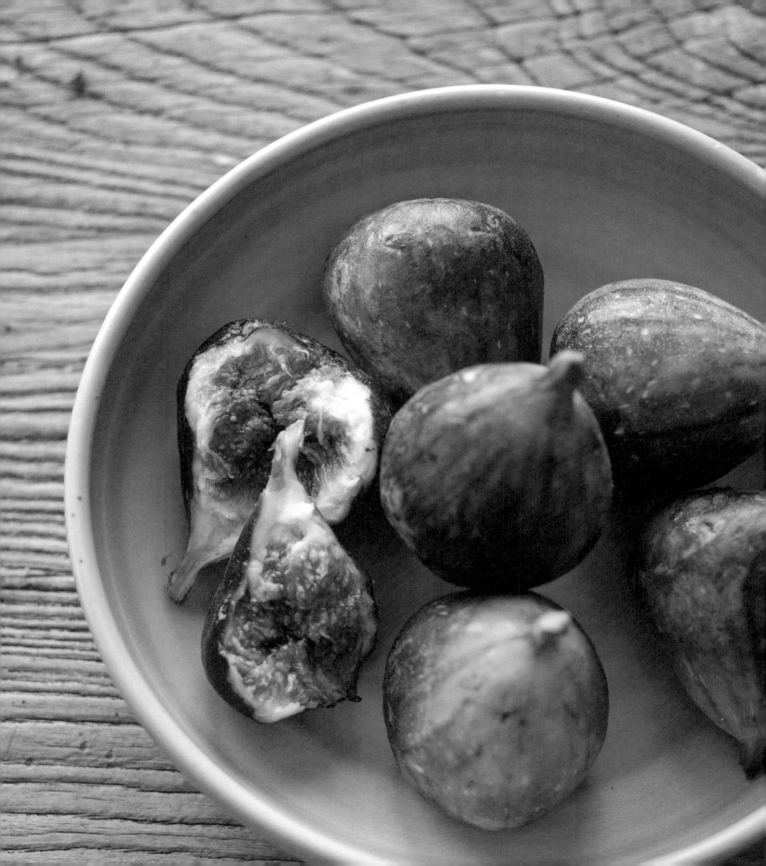

Recipe index

Subject index

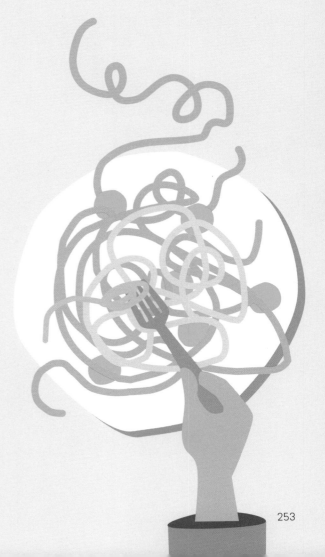

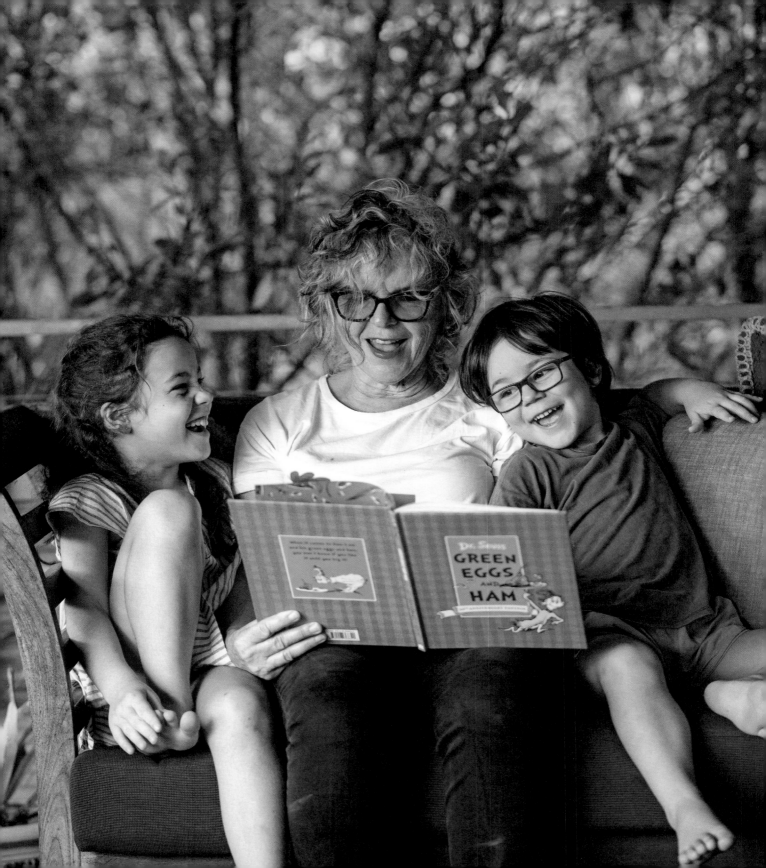

Acknowledgements

I'd like to thank some special people whose encouragement, support and talent have made this book a truly worthwhile project we can all be proud of. With their support I set out to make a difference, by making it easy for families to eat together and raise adventurous, healthy eaters.

First, thanks to my family: to my much better half, Martin; to our sons, Will and Eddie, and to their better halves, Jess and Sophia; and to my inspirational grandchildren, Eva, Noah and Cassius - thanks for being such constructive critics and lovers of good food.

Chefs Sarah Swan and Samantha Gowing, what fun we had in the kitchen and what great food you created - everyday delicious food for families!

For the photography, thank you to Alan Benson for your patience, creativity and the way you bring food to life, and also to Kristine Duran for the beautiful styling that inspires us to create beautiful meals for all the family.

For the fabulous baby bowls, glasses, trays and everything that makes it easy to feed your baby, thanks to the brilliant Australian homewares designers featured in the images in this book. We were so proud to work with you. Thanks to Love Mae, We Might Be Tiny, Nordlife, Bison Home, Mud Australia, The Clay Barn and Amelia Frank.

Thanks to Bay Grocer, Byron Bay for the great fresh fruit and veg in this book, and to the producers from the Northern Rivers of New South Wales for the delicious produce you grow every day. And to regenerative farmers the world over - thank you.

To everyone at Hardie Grant but especially Jane Willson, Loran McDougall and Ariana Klepac for your encouragement and support. Special thanks to the talented Emily O'Neill for the fabulous design and illustrations.

Published in 2021 by Hardie Grant Books,
an imprint of Hardie Grant Publishing

Hardie Grant Books (Melbourne)
Building 1, 658 Church Street
Richmond, Victoria 3121

Hardie Grant Books (London)
5th & 6th Floors
52-54 Southwark Street
London SE1 1UN

hardiegrantbooks.com

Green Eggs and Ham (slipcase edition) by Dr Seuss,
shown and referenced on pp. 76-7, published in 2019
by Harper Collins.

We Can All Eat That!
ISBN 978 1 74379 579 8

10 9 8 7 6 5 4 3 2 1

A catalogue record for this
book is available from the
National Library of Australia

Publishing Director: Jane Willson
Project Editor: Loran McDougall
Editor: Ariana Klepac
Design Managers: Jessica Lowe and Mietta Yans
Designer and illustrator: Emily O'Neill
Photographer: Alan Benson
Stylist: Kristine Duran
Production Manager: Todd Rechner

Colour reproduction by Splitting Image Colour Studio
Printed in China by Leo Paper Products LTD.

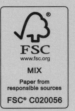

The paper this book is printed on is from
FSC®-certified forests and other sources.
FSC® promotes environmentally responsible,
socially beneficial and economically viable
management of the world's forests.

Disclaimer: The use of this book is at the sole risk of the
reader. Its content does not replace medical advice and is
not a substitution for a physician's advice for, or diagnosis
of, any health issue. The reader should regularly consult a
physician in relation to any health issues. The author and
publisher have no responsibility in relation to any adverse
effects arising from following any advice given in this book.
The reader accepts all risks and responsibility for losses,
damages, costs and other consequences resulting directly
or indirectly from using this book. To the maximum permitted
by law, the author and publisher exclude all liability to any
person arising directly or indirectly from using this book.

The author, Pam Brook, wrote this book with the latest
research available at the time of writing. While Dr Anne
Swain provided guidance, the author is responsible for
the content in this book.

Hardie Grant acknowledges the Traditional Owners of the
country on which we work, the Wurundjeri people of the
Kulin nation and the Gadigal people of the Eora nation, and
recognises their continuing connection to the land, waters
and culture. We pay our respects to their Elders past,
present and emerging.

'Pam Brook has managed to distil a relaxed, real-food approach into a user-friendly guide for new parents ... and finally! Recipes for tots that are more about what to pack in, rather than what to leave out.'

Alice Zaslavsky, author and presenter

'As a mother of five, I can attest that no matter how many times you've done it before, introducing new foods to your baby can be such a confusing time. This book offers straightforward advice and tips (and delicious recipes!) to help you navigate this period with ease and enjoyment.'

Courtney Adamo, author and founder of In The Loop

'A beautiful book that brings a calm and measured approach to establishing healthy lifetime eating habits, from the very youngest among us – and up. The gorgeous yet simple recipes are coupled with pragmatic, medically sound advice that helps navigate the often confusing messages, and pressures, surrounding food allergies and the best approach for introducing foods to babies and children.'

Pip Taylor, sports nutritionist